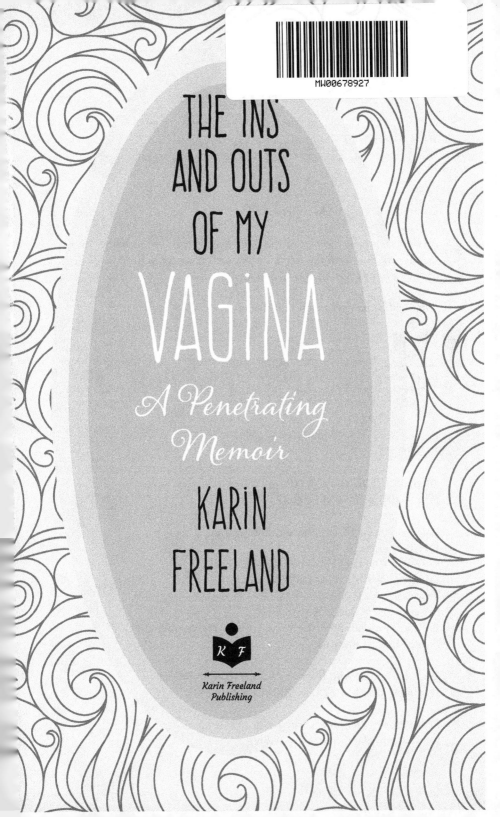

THE INS AND OUTS OF MY

VAGINA

A Penetrating Memoir

KARIN FREELAND

Karin Freeland
Publishing

Published by Karin Freeland Publishing

Karin Freeland
Publishing

Printed in the United States of America
10 9 8 7 6 5 4 3 2 1

eBook ISBN: 978-1-7923-7192-9
Print ISBN: 978-0-578-94998-7

Produced by GMK Writing and Editing, Inc.
Edited by Gary M. Krebs
Copyedited by Liz Crooks and EpsteinWords
Proofread by Liz Crooks and EpsteinWords
Text design and composition by Libby Kingsbury
Cover design by Libby Kingsbury
Back cover author photo by Yolanda Perez Photography LLC
Printed by IngramSpark

You can connect with Karin on Instagram @karinfreeland and on Facebook.com/KarinFreelandLifeCoaching.

Learn more about how Karin transforms women's lives at www.karinfreeland.com/life-coaching.

If someone asked me to pick out my own vagina's mug shot out of a lineup of vaginas, I'd be helpless. And probably concerned about what exactly my vagina had been doing that constituted a need for its own mug shot.

—*Jenny Lawson*, Let's Pretend This Never Happened: A Mostly True Memoir

To my loving—and very understanding—husband…
…who put aside his own reservations and supported me through the
entire process. You really are an amazing (and tolerant) man!
Thanks for loving me and V just the way we are.

To my boys…
…who are begging to read my work, because they are certain it's a real
gut-buster and can't figure out how I have so many stories about my
vagina. I hope you still want to be seen with me in public
if you read this someday.

To Peanut…
…you'll always be my first baby. I'm glad your memory will forever be
captured on these pages. My heart aches without your smiling face and
wagging tail around. What I wouldn't give for you to cock-block me
and Daddy one more time!

To all the people who contributed to my vagina trials and tribulations…
…you'll always have a special place in my heart.

I'd be remiss if I didn't also dedicate this book to V…
…after all, she's the reason there is a book in the first place. Thanks for
putting up with me. I can't think of a better partner in crime.

ACKNOWLEDGMENTS

To my parents...I used to force you to drop me off around the corner, so now it's your turn to be embarrassed of me. You're welcome! Thanks for supporting me in your own loving way.

To my sister...for always telling it to me like it is. You called out my writing when it was crap and made me work harder. Love you! You'll always be a driving force in my life and business.

To my editor, Gary M. Krebs...for helping me craft this story and truly bringing out the funny moments in my life. Your guidance and counsel have been a tremendous help. I could not have created this book without you.

To Chris Formant, my former boss and mentor...for introducing me to my editor. You didn't have to take my call or put your reputation on the line by sharing my idea with your network, but you did. Thank you for not hanging up on me as soon as I said I was writing a book about my vagina!

To my cousin, Bill Paggio...who was my fellow black sheep of the family as a teenager and and will forever be my "cool cousin." Thank you for being my original editor and helping me get the draft in good shape to be able to share it with others and secure a professional editor. Your praise motivated me like nothing else and I owe you lots of beer in return!

To my cousin, Nicole Lucciola...who spent countless hours reading my drafts and inspired me to keep going.

To my dear friend, Nina, from Real Talk with Nina...who gave me the confidence to take this book from my computer into the real world. Your constant support and motivation kept me going and I'm forever grateful.

To my former co-worker...who asked me point blank what I wanted to do before I died. That very question spurred me to pull this memoir off the figurative shelf and give it life. I might still be in Corporate America making PowerPoint presentations to justify my existence if it weren't for that question.

To the countless other people who have shown support and encouraged me along the way...you know who you are, and I love you to pieces!

CONTENTS

Part 4: Miami Heat

Part 5: Sexual Peaks and Valleys

Part 6: No Vacancy

Part 7: Clam-tastrophes

Part 8: The Final Curtain

To Womb It May Concern

We're about to become very intimate with one another—after all, this book is titled THE INS AND OUTS OF MY VAGINA. I hope you are ready for some gut-busting, jaw-dropping, mind-blowing mishaps and misadventures!

You are invited to take an intimate glimpse into my personal life: the sexy, the gross, the funny, and a lot more. I hope you can relate to it and, along the way, have a few laughs you can share with friends (and maybe siblings and other confidants as well). My intent is for this book to provide a sense of comfort and camaraderie for women twenty-one and up, although I know some teens will probably sneak peeks at the juicier bits (as will a few guys).

I wouldn't say that sharing these details of my life came easily. Believe it or not, I'm generally not this open with people, often covering up what's truly going on in my life. Growing up, my mom avoided conflict like the plague. That has certainly played a role in my life and impacted how I deal with challenging situations.

Many people have asked me, "How on earth did you come to write a book about your vagina?" First, I would tell you that this book is about so much more than my vagina. It's about growing up and going through puberty, learning to experiment and push your boundaries, finding love and creating life, and trying your damnedest to have an orgasm before you reach fifty. It just happens to be told through the lens (as it were) of my vagina.

It started out as a joke between my husband and me, while I was pregnant with our first child. My husband was always amazed at how clueless I was about how my vagina worked. In fact, it wasn't until I started writing this book that I realized a vagina and a vulva aren't the same thing! (I'll tell you all about the exact origin in Chapter Thirty, "All Lubed Up with Nowhere to Go," but, for now, let's just say it involves some olive oil and the female taint!)

Names have been changed to protect the identities of those included in the book. I realize that, while I find most of this hilarious, many of those who contributed to my vagina misadventures likely do not wish to be identified.

My goal for this book was not only self-discovery, but to provide support for other women who, like me, truly don't know their own respective vaginas.

In Vagina Solidarity,

Karin

Note: Throughout this book, you will read the word *vagina* quite a bit, including when I have conversations with her (referred to as V in much of the book). Please note that I have taken some creative liberties here. Despite the general use of the word *vagina* to refer to the whole of women's genital anatomy, this is actually incorrect. The vagina is the birth canal where babies come out and penises (and/or dildos) can go in. The *vulva* is the external portion of women's genital anatomy; it includes the inner lips, the vaginal opening, the *mons pubis*, and the external portion of the clitoris. Most of the nerve endings needed for women to orgasm are on the outside (the vulva), not the inside (the vaginal canal) of women's genitals. In fact, only about 4%-18% of women are capable of achieving an orgasm from penetration alone. When we refer to our entire genitals as a vagina, we are linguistically erasing the part of ourselves that gives us the most pleasure (Mintz, 2017). The language I use in this book is for comedic purposes only, not to suggest any type of erasure.

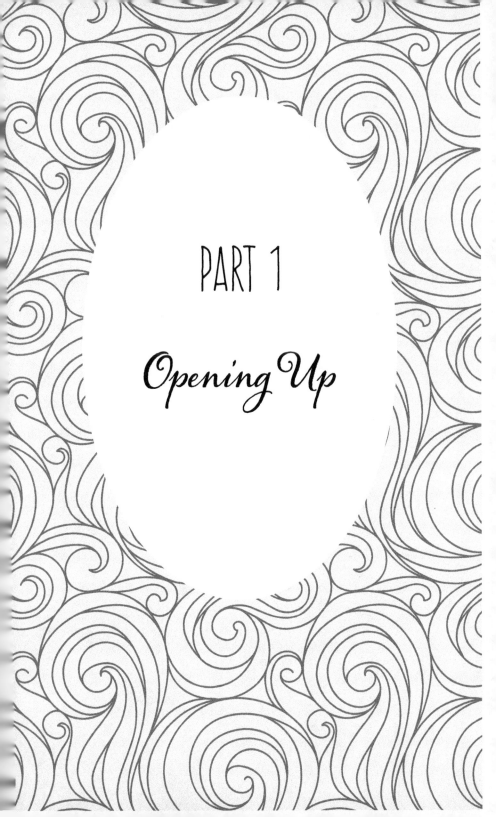

PART 1

Opening Up

*M*y adolescence may be summed up in a few words: *awkward, clunky, tragic.*

Awkward on account of my looks. To begin with, I spent an extra month in my mom's vagina avoiding entrance into the world. Apparently, I've always had a thing for vaginas. That additional time in her birth canal proved costly for me, as it resulted in a deviated septum for life. My nose was so mis-formed that the doctor instructed my mom to massage my nose back into place for several months.

I wasn't exactly beauty pageant material for other reasons as well. My ears stuck straight out of the sides of my head. They weren't big *per se*, but I hadn't grown into them, either. Lastly, my two front teeth had a gap between them that made me look like Bucky Beaver.

Clunky because of my personality. The Energizer Bunny had nothing on me. I could talk your ear off with zero effort. I had a lot to say and wanted to make sure everyone heard me. When it came to boys, I had no idea how to act around them. My personality only intensified, and I found myself stuck in the friend zone with boys through elementary school. Labeled a prude, I vowed to do anything it would take to change that over the next dozen years.

Tragic in the dramatic *woe-is-me* sense. Although I didn't see it at the time, I had a relatively normal upbringing in the grand scheme of things. But there were a few notable unusual experiences that shaped my journey to womanhood, which I'll share with you now.

ONE

Discovering My Lady Parts

My journey into understanding my womanhood began on a hot summer weekend in June. I lived with my parents and sister, Debra, in a modest house that was nestled in a quaint development, which was still being expanded. We were your typical Upstate New York, middle-class suburban family. If you've never been to Upstate, think rolling hills, winding back roads, and strip malls. It was the mid-1980s, so pigtails and ruffled-sleeve bathing suits were all the rage. I was five years old, maybe six. I was swimming in our circular-shaped, above-ground pool in the backyard, cooling off from the hot summer sun. I loved nothing more than to spend the entire day in the water to the point of turning my fingers and toes all pruny.

"Let's make a whirlpool!" I shouted to my dad.

"Okay," he replied. "Follow me."

He began to walk briskly in one direction with my sister on his back. She wore floaties to prevent her slipping away from him. Both of us were like fish in the water, though. We might as well have been born in the pool.

My mom stood by, watching from the deck. Unless it was over 95 degrees outside, she rarely entered the pool. I can't say I blame her; I've become the same way as an adult.

I giggled as I tried to walk in the same direction as my dad. Being vertically challenged (in other words, short), I had to use my feet to push off the pool floor. My head bobbed under water each time. I'd come back up giggling and gasping for air, as my dad passed me on his way around the pool. Before long, the force of the whirlpool had taken shape. I could now lie on my back and float around the pool in circles. It was a good thing, too, because I was getting winded from trying to create the whirlpool. It felt good to relax in the motion of the water.

Suddenly, I found I had to relieve myself. Since my parents were adamantly opposed to anyone peeing in the pool, I stuck my hand out to grab the pool ladder as I floated by it. I used my tiny arms to pull myself out of the whirlpool and exit the water. I snatched my towel to pat myself dry and ran into the house. Having done a subpar job of drying myself off, I ran upstairs while still half-wet and dripping water across the dining room carpet and on the stairwell.

"Don't run! You're going to slip and fall!" my mom shouted from the patio.

I rushed into the bathroom. Squeezing my legs together, I slammed the door and hopped toward the toilet. Heeding my mom's warning, I tried not to slip. The tile floor felt cold on my wet feet as I made my way to the bowl.

It was no secret around school that boys have penises and girls have vaginas. As I sat on the porcelain toilet of our middle-class suburban house with my blue bathing suit dangling from my feet, I began to check out my vagina. You can imagine my dismay when I discovered that…I had a penis!

Well, let me explain.

I had not seen a penis up until that time—remember: I was only five or six—so it wasn't as if I had any idea of what I was looking at as I peered down between my legs. *Something* was sticking out. Something pink and roundish. I poked at it.

"Hmn," I said to myself. "What can this be? I've never seen this before."

I finished urinating and tugged my wet bathing suit back on. I rushed downstairs to my Mom without having washed my hands.

"Mom! Mom! I need to show you something. It's an emergency," I called to her as I stepped out onto the patio.

I was still panting, with a dripping wet bathing suit, as I placed my hands on my knees and looked up at her. The sun shone right in my eyes, causing me to squint.

"What is it, Karin?"

"I have a *penis*!" I shouted for the entire world to hear.

Before she could respond, I lowered my ruffled bathing suit strap and revealed my discovery.

I don't remember the exact words she used, but I do recall her reaction; it was somewhere between insane laughter and utter disgust. Mainly, though, she probably felt embarrassed, as our neighbors peeked across our patio to get a look at the girl with the male organ.

My mother grabbed my arm and dragged me back inside the house. She reassured me that I *do not* have a penis. She explained to me that lady parts consist of a lot more than just "holes to pee from." They feature "other things," one of which I had mistaken for a penis. I would learn all about them when I was older—*much* older. Obviously, my mom's detailed explanation cleared things right up for me. I went back to swimming feeling relieved I hadn't sprouted a penis overnight.

You might be asking yourself, "How does she mistake a clitoris for a penis? Is hers so gigantic?"

No. Mine has always been normal size. At least I *think* it is (and was). Then again, how would I know the difference? Even if I did, I can't see any possible benefit to it. To this day, I have never heard of a guy looking for a woman with an abnormally large clit. But, if he's out there, I might just be his dream girl.

TWO

Twat Was That?

FACT: IT'S POSSIBLE FOR A FETUS TO MASTURBATE IN THE WOMB. I don't have any idea of what a fetus could possibly be fantasizing about. If I happen to have performed the act myself at that time, I can't say I recall any specific images.

Don't worry, I won't probe any further into womb masturbation. Instead, let's fast-forward a year or two to my first solo sexual experience that I can recall. Let's say I was around age seven. It's not as if I was keeping a diary about these things at the time, so I can't be one hundred percent certain.

My mom was giving Debra a bath, and I was up next. She asked me to wait nearby, so I got ready—stark naked—while the tub drained. Apparently, I didn't have a modest bone in my body as a youngster—a quality that would gradually change.

During my wait, I happened upon a sleeping bag on the floor of my parents' bedroom, probably a remnant of a Girl Scout trip. I figured that I might as well bide my time in the sleeping bag until it was my turn to bathe.

I slid inside the material and zipped myself up tight. I buried my head within. It felt like nighttime, even though the sun was shining through my parents' large picture window. The hardwood floor underneath me was unforgiving. I wished I had a pillow but couldn't be bothered to get up and find one. I was wiggling my legs around to situate myself when I was overcome by a certain sensation that sprang forth between my legs and rose up throughout my body.

My head began to spin with thoughts: *What is this? I've never felt anything like it before. Is it getting hot in here? Maybe I should stick my head out and get some air? No, I kind of like it, whatever it is.*

I squeezed my legs harder together. The intensity of the sensation increased.

How am I making this happen? Is it magic? I hope bath time never comes....

Does anyone know what I'm doing in here? Why do I feel like I'm doing something terribly wrong?

At the same time, it was such a wonderful feeling. Moments passed, during which time I felt like I had disappeared into another universe. I wanted to remain in this sleeping bag forever with my legs clenched tight. I reached a point where I couldn't squeeze any harder, but the feeling lingered. I had no idea what my body was trying to achieve. Butterflies filled my stomach. My head became dizzy.

"Karin, come on, it's your turn!" my mom shouted from the bathroom.

Her voice rang in my ears like a jet breaking the sound barrier. I didn't want to budge, but I had already been disturbed and the blissful moment had dissipated.

"*Karin!*" she repeated.

I released my legs and unzipped the sleeping bag. Just as my reddened face popped out, Debra whizzed by draped in her towel. I wrestled out of the sleeping bag and forced myself to my feet while trying to keep my legs as close together as possible. I waltzed, somewhat shamefully, into the bathroom.

What have I just done?

I wondered if anyone could tell if something was different about me based on my appearance. I wiggled past my mother and plunked myself in the warm, bubbly water. She poured water over my head and began lathering baby shampoo into my hair. Everything seemed perfectly normal; she didn't reveal a trace of being onto me and, in fact, hummed a tune from the musical *Cats*. How fitting!

I lay in bed that evening and stared at the ceiling with only a glimmer of light shining on my bed from the hallway. I wondered if I could recreate what had happened in the sleeping bag. I wanted to try...but I was petrified.

What if I cause that part of my body to pop off?

And what if...God already knows I'm doing this? Is it a sin? Am I going to be allowed into heaven?

The fear of being caught by my mother and cast into hell didn't deter my curiosity. It wasn't long before I began to lock myself in my room and conduct mini-discovery sessions on my body. Night or day, whenever my family members were occupied, I would squirrel away in my room and experiment. Although I perpetually feared getting exposed, the temptation of pleasure always outweighed the risk.

And yet...even though I enjoyed the self-gratification, I did not experience the ultimate pleasure. Not that I could possibly have known what *that* was at the time but, of course, eventually I would learn what I had been missing...

The Big O: the bane of my existence.

THREE

Bushwhacked

Let's face it: When you are an adult, pubes suck! Shaving them, waxing them, seeing them jut out of your white bathing suit, getting them lodged in the teeth or throat while performing oral stimulation….

What's the point of them? They don't even keep a vagina warm in the winter.

Women spend thousands of dollars each year removing pubic hair. *No one* wants pubes as an adult.

And yet…when I was in sixth grade and the other girls in my class were getting their pubes, I desperately longed for those short and curlies! I prayed to God every night to bestow a few strands upon me down there, just to give an indication that I was becoming a woman. It didn't feel like a lot to ask. It wasn't as if I was asking for world peace.

Morning after morning when I awoke, I peeked inside my underwear to see if anything had sprouted down there. Each time, I would be met with utter disappointment.

Flashback to a sleepover…

The year: 1991.

The setting: a dimly lit, finished basement in my friend Jenna's house.

The cast: ten girls from my elementary school, including myself.

Bowls of chips and pretzels were scattered around the room, along with a few two-liter bottles of soda. (We were too young to care about calories or sugar intake.)

We had already watched a movie and done each other's makeup. It was nearing 1:00 AM and there was only one thing left to do....

"Who wants to play Truth or Dare?" a girl named Tina asked the group.

"Yeah, I do!" someone chimed in.

"Me too," followed another.

That was all it took. We had a consensus and began to play Truth or Dare. The game began innocently enough, as it always does.

TRUTH: *Do you like Johnny?*

DARE: *Prank call—Brian.*

TRUTH: *Would you rather kiss Todd or Chris?*

These are easy; they're throwing out softballs. This is getting boring, even for a sixth grader.

In those days, when you brought so many girls together, things were bound to take a turn for the worse at some point. Suddenly, without any warning, the first real zinger shot across the basement...

DARE: *Show us your boobs.*

Then the second...

DARE: *Moon us!*

Next...it was my turn. I was on the receiving end and couldn't back down. The tension mounted as the group of girls focused solely on me.

My inner voice began to shout: *Don't say DARE! Don't say DARE!*

I could feel the girls silently willing me into uttering the one word I didn't want to say. My resolve was weakening; I knew I was going to buckle at any moment.

ME (squinting, in an attempt to look tough): *Dare!*

DARE: *Show us your pubes!*

Damn it! Of all DARES, why did I have to get *this one?* My worst nightmare was coming to fruition. I was the shortest one in the group, and the girls had already deduced that there was some correlation between height and time of puberty. They had conspired together, specifically choosing this DARE because they believed I had a barren desert down there.

Nevertheless, I received the challenge and had to face up to it. Karin Freeland never backed down from a DARE!

I stood up, revealing my New Kids on the Block tee-shirt and striped granny panties from JCPenney. My bare feet felt cold and numb on the tiled basement floor. My cheeks turned beet red as I tugged down my underwear.

The room became silent. The other girls gawked, open-mouthed in amazement. Without any warning at all, a bush snapped out of my panties like a tree branch that had been pulled back and then released.

I quietly celebrated in my mind: *I have pubes—lots of them! I've been vindicated!*

They were curly, they were thick, and they were glorious. They had seemed to grow in overnight but it was probably closer to two months. A small fly could have gotten lost in that forest. Despite all of my fears of being a late developer, all signs were now to the contrary: My vagina had miraculously knitted itself a fur coat.

FOUR

Aunt Flow Pays Her First Visit

JUNIOR HIGH SCHOOL WAS AN INCREDIBLY AWKWARD TIME FOR ME, as it is for most kids entering their teen years. Outside of my early physical development, it was not a sexually active time by any stretch of the imagination. (Perhaps the glasses and retainer had something to do with it?)

Now, just as sprouting pubic hair is a rite of passage for a girl, so is getting her first period. This one is bigger, though—far more significant. Technically, once a girl experiences her first menstrual cycle, she is a woman. I longed for the day when I would get my period but, like many things that seem cool when you're a little kid, it's much less appealing when it actually happens.

I was twelve years old at the time. I vividly remember that Tuesday morning and having been awakened at 5:20 AM by the bleeping of my alarm. My bedroom was pitch black, except for a sliver of light that peeked through the crack in the door. My hand reached over to slap the snooze button. I rolled over to get another ten minutes of sleep. When the alarm sounded again, I bolted out of bed and grabbed a towel from the hall closet before entering the bathroom. I flicked on the light and made sure both doors were locked, since my parents had their own entrance to the bathroom from their bedroom. I was less concerned about one of them coming in than I was about my sister entering uninvited.

I removed my oversized tee-shirt and threw it in a corner on the floor. I turned on the shower, so it would warm up before I got in. Standing only in my underwear, I pulled out the scale. I stepped on it to check my weight: eighty-one pounds. I nodded in agreement with the scale.

By now, the water in the shower stall was warm enough for me to step in. After carefully testing the temperature with my toes, I let the water spray over my hair and grabbed a bottle of Nexxus shampoo. Having long hair required that I apply just the right squeeze of shampoo as if were an art form. Too much, and it would take forever to rinse out; too little, and there would be no lather and I'd have greasy hair for the next two days. With my eyes closed, I lathered every strand before rinsing out the suds backwards down the drain. Once I was sure the shampoo was gone, my eyes flickered open through the water.

I happened to be looking down at my feet when something strange caught my eyes and made me gasp. Red water was pooling in the bathtub, along with the clear droplets.

Oh crap, I'm bleeding! What the hell is going on? I didn't cut myself. I haven't even started shaving my legs yet.

Then it dawned on me....

Is this what I think it is? It must be. This is the exact moment I've been waiting for. I've got my period—finally! It's official: At the ripe old age of twelve, I am becoming a woman.

The more I thought about it, however, the less exciting this situation seemed to be....

Okay, what now? Oh, this is pretty gross. How long is this blood going to keep streaming out of me?

Reality began to sink in, as I struggled to figure out how I was going to step out of the shower, leave the bathroom, and get my mom to help me without making a mess everywhere and tipping off other family members. I certainly did not want my dad to know.

I reached for a bar of soap and lathered up a washcloth. As I cleaned myself off, it struck me that the timing of this event couldn't have been better. I'd had nightmares about it happening in class and staining my jeans. It would have been mortifying facing the jeers of my classmates as I dashed out to the girls' room.

Instead, I had all the privacy in the world. I thought about whom I was going to tell when I arrived at school. I couldn't wait to share the good news with my closest friends. I would finally be part of the club, which has a lifetime membership. (I had no idea about menopause; that shocker would come later!)

At last, the blood seemed to subside as my shower drew to a close. I grabbed my towel and dried myself off as I normally would. I was about to toss away the towel when I saw crimson stains all over it.

Ugh, no. I thought it was done. Great. What am I going to do with this towel? Mom is going to kill me.

I couldn't stand there any longer. I needed something to soak up the blood—*and fast.* I ran to the cabinet under the sink, where I began tossing aside hairsprays and curlers. Buried in the back was a stash of my mom's maxi pads. My jaw dropped as I pulled one out of the box.

Wow, this thing is massive! But it ought to do the trick.

I kept checking between my legs to see if more blood was dripping out. I took the maxi pad and haphazardly placed it against my vagina. I poked my head through the bathroom door to get a lay of the land. I hadn't brought any clothes into the bathroom with me; I only had this bloody towel.

My dad was downstairs with his back to the stairwell. My mom and sister were still in their respective beds.

Phew!

This was my chance to make a run for it without being spotted.

I made my move and streaked through the hallway, all the while holding the maxi pad in place. This marked the first time I had to MacGyver a sanitary product—but it would not be the last.

I arrived safely in my room, locking the door behind myself. Afraid of dislodging the maxi pad from its place, I held it tightly as I hobbled to my dresser. I was still mostly wearing granny panties in seventh grade, and instinctively grabbed the oldest pair I could find so I wouldn't ruin any good ones. I gingerly stepped into the underwear, trying to maintain my balance while clenching the maxi pad tightly against my bleeding vagina. Once the panties were up high enough, I realized I had to remove the strip to reveal the sticky part of the pad and affix it to my underwear. I struggled to dig my nail underneath the edge to get the peel started. My nails kept losing their grip; the plastic slipped and got stuck back to the adhesive.

I attempted it again and again. Sweat poured off my forehead.

This period business is hard work.

Frustrated, I moved the maxi pad away from my body and tore the strip off in one manic motion. I prayed that the blood wouldn't drip onto my unprotected underwear or onto the bedroom floor. Luckily, I was able to situate everything without a hitch.

Okay. Now what?

I looked around my room for dark jeans. No such luck. It was 1993, and the only thing in sight was my light acid wash jeans. They would have to do. I wiggled them up over my hips.

Whoa, this is really uncomfortable. I feel like I'm wearing a diaper. Is this really what it's like to be a woman?

I hauled on my pink cotton bra. It was my favorite, and I secretly hoped it would make me feel better. I faced away from my mirror and twisted my neck to look at my butt.

Is anyone going to figure out what I'm wearing underneath these jeans?

I walked a few steps back and forth. The maxi pad didn't seem visible, but it felt like I had cotton balls soaked in sticky honey down there.

In order to ensure I wouldn't be exposed, I rummaged through my closet for a shirt that was long enough to cover my butt. My favorite oversized green tee-shirt would do.

At around 6:30, I slinked out of my room and headed downstairs for breakfast.

Perfect: Dad is back upstairs getting ready for work.

I was thankful to avoid conversation with anyone. I emptied some Lucky Charms into a bowl, followed by a generous portion of milk. I always ate the non-marshmallow part of the cereal first, because I loved to drink the marshmallow-soaked milk at the end. My mind wandered as I sat at the table eating and reading the back of the box.

I'm a woman now. Should I really be eating Lucky Charms? That's so childish of me. Raisin Bran, or even Wheaties, would be a more mature choice. That's it. Starting tomorrow, I will only eat cereal that is appropriate for a woman.

Before I knew it, the time had arrived for me to head to the bus stop. Before leaving, I tiptoed into my mom's room. The room was dark, and she was sleeping cozily under the covers on this winter morning. I stepped around to her side of the bed and leaned my head in close.

"Mom," I whispered. "I got my period this morning."

Her eyes snapped open: "You *did?*"

Perhaps in shock that her baby girl was growing up before her eyes, she focused on practicality rather than celebration. "Did you know where my pads were?"

"Yeah, I found them."

"Okay," she processed. "Well, make sure you bring some extra in your backpack, honey."

Right. Of course. I hadn't thought about that.

"How many do I need—two? Ten?"

"Why don't you bring four, just to be safe."

"Four. Got it. Thanks. Bye."

I hugged her and raced toward the bathroom.

"Love you," she called out to me.

Four. I need to get four....

I couldn't control my smile as I hurried into the bathroom, grabbed four maxi pads, and stuffed them in my backpack. I scurried down the steps and burst out the front door. I stood proud and tall as I skipped—well, more like waddled—to the bus stop. I reached it just as the bus was arriving and cut in front of one of the boys. I thought I heard a snicker but didn't pay it any mind. I climbed aboard and made my way down the crowded aisle, taking care not to trip over the legs and knees cluttering the way. I found a seat next to my friend Adeline. I was bursting at the seams to reveal my exciting—yet somewhat traumatizing—news. I was about to whisper in her ear when a voice echoed through the bus.

"Freeland got her period!" shouted a boy named Ben who was a few grades ahead of me. His only discernible physical characteristic was a head of dreadfully curly hair. Ben was the bus terror, always picking on someone. I couldn't stand seeing him under normal circumstances but, on this day, I longed to turn him upside down and use his head as a mop on the bus floor.

Oh my gosh—how did he know? Had I bled through the pad already? I'm totally screwed. Ruined for life.

My pulse raced. Everything started to go blurry.

Please, God, let me wake up from this nightmare.

I had no choice but to fight back. Denial seemed like my best—and only—strategy at this point.

"What are you talking about? I did not," I protested.

"Yeah?" he laughed. "Then why do you have a month's worth of pads in your backpack?"

Busted. All of my efforts to conceal my state had failed miserably.

I glanced down and realized that my bag hadn't been zipped all the way; a pad jutted out of the open space. I welled up in tears. The entire bus was now well aware that I had gotten my period.

Chants of *Freeland got her period* rippled throughout the bus.

My upset turned to rage. While I'd heard the *f*-word a few times, I rarely spoke it myself. In that moment, I became possessed.

"Fuck you!" I exclaimed.

Freeland got her period, Freeland got her period, Freeland got her period....

I buried my face in my lap in shame.

"Everybody sit down and shut up!" intervened Mandy, the

middle-aged bus driver. "I don't want to hear another word about anybody's period."

I'd regarded Mandy as being somewhat rough around the edges—I suppose she had to be managing all of these rowdy kids every day—but she revealed a softer side when she winked at me in the rearview mirror as if to say, *I've got your back.*

The next fifteen minutes in that seat were the longest of my life.

Maybe I could call my mom and have her pick me up from the nurse's office? Yes, that's it—it's worth a shot.

My *Carrie* moment had happened, and I needed to stop this right in its tracks. If my mom were to pick me up, I figured, the headline of my period would become old news before lunch time.

My mom understood completely and brought me home. I spent the remainder of the day binge-eating Doritos and watching soap operas.

The following morning, I was again prepared with the maxi pads, but concealed them better in the backpack and made sure it was zipped up tight this time. I took my seat on the bus next to Adeline and held my breath. After a few minutes, I scanned around: No one was paying the slightest attention to me, including Ben. I was off the hook.

Adeline elbowed me. I turned toward her grinning, knowing face. This said it all. My vagina wasn't going to ruin my life after all!

FIVE

Panty Hot Potato

I WAS EXCITED WHEN I WAS INVITED TO MY FIRST BOY-GIRL POOL party of junior high, especially since a few of my close friends were attending—as well the guy I had been eyeing. I made sure to RSVP right away and counted down the days leading up to the party.

The day finally arrived. I thanked my lucky stars that I didn't have my period. That would have been the worst, I thought, to deal with tampons or pads at a pool party. Unsure if it would be warm enough to swim or if I was comfortable enough to wear my bathing suit in front of all these guys, I packed my bathing suit and a towel in a small duffel bag.

"Karin, we need to leave in five minutes," my mom called out. "Make sure you use the restroom before we go."

No matter how old I get, Mom still reminds me to use the restroom before we go anywhere.

I took the opportunity to pee, as suggested. While seated, I couldn't help but take a look downward at my underwear. I gasped in disgust.

Yuck. Discharge. What the hell is the stuff, anyway? Does it serve a purpose other than staining my underwear?

What if this happens at the party and I have to change into my bathing suit?... I got it! I'll put one of those thin pantyliners on.

My mom happened to keep a stash under the sink. I had used them from time to time, but now I thought they would come in handy. I completed my business and duck-walked over to the sink with my shorts and underwear around my knees. While in this position, I couldn't pick my feet up that high and my left foot snagged on the small carpet in front of the sink. My body tilted forward; fortunately, I regained my balance on the counter before my face struck the floor tiles. I exhaled and rummaged through the contents under the sink.

That was a close one. Not only is discharge gross; it's also dangerous.

I found a box of liners, yanked one out, and ripped off the backing, exposing the adhesive. I attached it to my underwear. I stood there for a moment while debating whether or not I should pack a second one. Ultimately, I made the decision not to, which would prove to be socially fatal.

Fifteen minutes later, I was entering the party and handing a wrapped gift to the birthday girl. She thanked me and showed me to her room. "Everyone is throwing their stuff on my floor, so just leave your bag in here," she instructed me.

"Okay, cool," I replied.

"We're playing manhunt. Want to be on my team?"

"Sure! Is Henry here yet?" I asked.

Henry was the boy I had been crushing on in band. I played the clarinet; poorly, but I played.

"Yeah…why? You like him or something?"

"Oh no," I lied. "Just need to tell him something about band practice the other day."

She seemed to buy my story and trotted through the house back to the patio. An hour later everything was going fine. We played manhunt and devoured some pizza. I only had one slice because I knew swimming would be next, and I didn't want to seem bloated.

"Who's ready to go swimming?" my friend's mom invited.

Everyone shouted affirmations and we were provided with

instructions on where to change. All of the girls were led to my friend's room.

Wait? Are we all getting undressed in front of each other? No, no, no. This won't work. First of all, I am not getting naked in front of these girls. Second, I have a pantyliner on. There is no chance I'm going to change into my bikini bottoms with a dirty pantyliner on.

I wanted to crawl under a rock. My skin heated up. I needed a game plan, stat.

I know—I'll say I have to use the bathroom and change in there. Yep, that's all I've got.

I fumbled through my bag to buy some time as the other girls stripped down and put their suits on. Apparently, they weren't as modest as I was. A few of the girls exited to the pool, which was my cue to make a break for the bathroom.

I shouldn't have been surprised by what I found: That pesky discharge was still oozing out. And I had been too dumb to take an extra pantyliner.

Damn. I knew I should have trusted my gut.

My first thought was to rectify the problem later on by stuffing my panties with tissues. Then it occurred to me that this would be problematic if we were to play a game like manhunt again; the tissues might fall out of my shorts while I was running.

It was pretty clear this soiled pantyliner would have to make do for the rest of the party. I left it on my underwear but wiped it off a bit before balling up the panties and sticking them in the pocket of my shorts so no one would see them. I finished putting on my suit and picked up my clothes. I could hear the screams of fun coming from the pool and wanted to hurry up and get out there. I scurried to my friend's room and dropped my clothes in a pile on my duffel bag, my tee-shirt positioned right on top of my shorts. I was out the door and splashing in the pool with the other kids in no time.

We played chicken, Marco Polo, and dunk the person you have a crush on. I was particularly good at the last game and wasted no time dunking Henry over and over again. I remained in the pool after most of the others left and went inside to change. I was having so much fun that I didn't want to get out of the water.

When my hands were sufficiently pruned, I decided to climb out and dry off so I could have some cake. I grabbed my towel from a lounge chair, dabbed myself off, and wrapped it around my body. Once certain I was drip-free, I stepped into the house and through the short hallway toward my friend's bedroom. I heard quite a ruckus going on—girls' voices and swirling laughter—but didn't think much of it, until…I opened the door and looked inside.

My smile dwindled. My heart sank.

My duffel bag—as well as everything I had carefully arranged—was in disarray. My shirt had been tossed on the floor, several feet away from my stuff. The shorts? *Gone.*

My eyes darted to and fro among the three girls jumping around on the bed. They were tossing an object around while spewing out commentary.

"*Ewww*, gross!"

"Hot potato—not mine!"

"Yuck—stained underwear!"

"Whose are these?!"

I knew right away what the hot potato was—and *whose* it was: my panties.

Oh my gosh, what do I do? Do I pretend they aren't mine? Do I ask for my underwear back and hope they don't tell every single person at our school about the incident?

I mumbled, "Oh…those are mine," but no one could hear me over the yelling and high-pitched giggling. Suddenly, the underwear went flying through the air and landed on the carpet right in front of me. All of the girls stared at me.

I had to react, one way or the other. "Gross!" I recoiled, playing along. "Don't throw them at me!"

My acting must have been at least somewhat convincing, as two bored girls bounced off the bed and left to join the main party.

Luckily, the others followed. I felt a brief moment of relief, but I wasn't quite off the hook. One girl, Dana, lingered. Undoubtedly, she had been the ringleader of the game.

The tension mounted as she stared right at me with an expression indicating she knew the underwear was mine. I felt mortified. I envisioned her—forgive the pun—leaking this out to the entire junior high school. I froze in place while waiting for her to react.

Then, for no apparent reason, she wordlessly rose and left the room. How could I have been blessed by such good fortune? Stunned, I remained in place with my contaminated panties on the floor in front of me.

Oh my God, now's my chance before someone barges in. I have to move fast.

I snatched up my underwear, grabbed my clothes, and rushed to the bathroom to change. I removed my bathing suit, pulled on my disgusting underwear, and tugged on my shorts. In hindsight, throwing out the liner and getting my underwear dirty from the discharge would probably have been a more hygienic (and less embarrassing) decision, but my brain wasn't fully developed. That's my story and I'm sticking to it.

I rejoined the party. No one said a single word about my "hot potato." I had averted disaster, unscathed—at least in terms of public humiliation. However, my perceived vaginal dysfunction from the event lingered long afterwards. I remained convinced I was the only woman who suffered from discharge and/or didn't know how to adequately prevent it.

Years later, I was reminded of the incident—and provided some solace—while watching *Amy Schumer: Live at the Apollo* on HBO. Schumer opened her routine by offering two New Year's resolutions. The second went like this: "No. 2 was to this year just once take off a pair of underwear and make it not look like I blew my nose in it."

As long as we have vaginas, that is a resolution that will never come true—for Amy or me!

SIX

Tongue Tango

GROWING UP, THERE WAS ONE THING I LOVED TO DO: ATTEND FRIDAY night high school football games. Everything about them excited me: the lights on the field; the players in their uniforms; the cheerleaders on the track; the groups of friends hanging out under the bleachers. I can still recall the smell and feel of the crisp fall air on my face and hear the sounds of the marching band in my head.

Anyone who knew me back in eighth grade will remember how much I loved my Champion sweatshirts. I had one for every day of the week, but the purple one was my favorite. Naturally, I wore it for game night when I expected to kiss Carter, my boyfriend of three days. (Long-term relationships were a challenge for me.) Maybe it had something to do with my style or lack thereof? Back then I always had my hair in a ponytail because I didn't do "sexy," I did "cute." For some reason, all of my jeans ended up being high waters and, since I was scared of my boobs showing, my shirts were three sizes too large. I wouldn't develop any fashion sense until much later on.

All night I engaged in a cat-and-mouse game to avoid Carter, because that's what you do when you're totally awkward and afraid to kiss someone. At halftime, I stood near the snack stand where it was most crowded and I would be "safe" from his advances. My friend

Adeline and a few others stood by my side to keep watch. When any of us spotted him closing in, we would dart through the crowd to a new location. The more I ran and hid, the harder he pursued. Clearly, he enjoyed playing the role of cat as much as I did the mouse.

I made my way around the corner of the bleachers. They towered over my head and shielded the pavement from any light.

Natasha broke the silence. "I don't know what you're so worried about, Karin," she scoffed. "You know I've already been to third base. It's no big deal."

The girls huddled with me in a tight circle as Natasha went on to describe how she had let a guy finger her.

Gross! How could she have allowed him to do this to her?

That was the least of it. Another friend, Marlena, one-upped her: "That's nothing. Dave ate me out last weekend."

"What does *that* mean?" I asked, bewildered.

A few girls looked at me like I was a moron.

How am I supposed to know about such things? I don't have older siblings to ruin my innocence.

Marlena had no qualms about educating me: "He went down on me. You know, he put his mouth on my crotch…licked it…and stuff."

"While you were naked?" I asked.

"Yep, *naked.*"

The girls giggled at the news, but I didn't consider it amusing. I needed a spatula to scrape my jaw off the pavement.

Ew, no way! I will never let someone do that to me! I mean…I PEE from there. Why would someone ever want to lick me where I pee! No thanks!

Suddenly, I felt a hand on my back. Startled, I flipped around to see who was there. I let out a gasp: Carter stood right in front of me, blocking my path.

"I've been looking all over for you," he said in a domineering voice.

"Oh yeah? Well, looks like you found me," I teasingly replied, trying to conceal my nervousness.

Shit. Shit. Shit. Maybe I could fake a heart attack.

We stared wordlessly at each other as the sound of the cowbell rang in our ears. Before I could break our stalemate, he wrapped his arms around me and lifted me off the ground. His arms drew me in ever closer as my feet dangled in mid-air like spaghetti. I was a prisoner in his arms, helpless. His face approached mine and his tongue plunged into my mouth without warning.

Whoa—tongue?

My mind raced to figure out how I should respond. I tapped into the most respected, reputable source of information I could think of: *Seventeen* magazine. The writers and editors were the real deal— true experts, right? I recalled an article in which they suggested the exploration of our boyfriends' mouths using our tongues.

My tongue flew around in his mouth like the arm of a hand mixer, dodging his and seeking to explore every inch of his mouth. It felt nice, but deep down I knew I wasn't doing something right; "turbo tongue" could not have been what the editors at *Seventeen* had in mind.

Meanwhile, I couldn't tell if my eyes were open or shut; all I saw was darkness and stars. I was flooded with thoughts from a year earlier at my first boy-girl Halloween party where I was taught how to kiss by two friends:

"Have you ever kissed a boy before, Karin?" my friend Natasha probed.

"Well, no, not on the lips. What do I do?"

I was desperate for answers. It felt like my life depended on it.

"Don't worry. It's easy. I'll show you," Natasha volunteered.

Natasha took a pillow and brought it toward her face. Closing her eyes ever so gently, she puckered her lips, pressed them against the pillow and, like in a slow-motion movie scene, parted her lips as she pulled back. She looked so pretty kissing that pillow. No wonder all the boys liked her so much.

She continued the lesson: "It's easier if you practice on your hand. Come on, try it. Like this."

Natasha separated her lips and began licking the back of her hand while making kissing noises. My jaw hit the bed.

Whoa, is that a French kiss?

First, there was no way I was going to stick my tongue in a boy's mouth. Second, she looked ridiculous.

And yet…here I was with my tongue in a boy's mouth! Did I look ridiculous, too?

I emerged from my blackout newly aware of what I was doing and what had been happening around us. I'd been oblivious to the group of boys and girls who were counting the number of seconds Carter and I had been kissing.

"Five, six, seven…."

Great. We're on full display.

I pulled away from Carter's embrace. My feet finally hit the ground. The kiss itself wasn't so scary, after all, but my cheeks were beet red in embarrassment. I flashed him a smile and scurried to the safety of my friends.

"Your feet weren't even on the floor," one friend marveled. "We thought he was going to eat your face!"

That went well…not!

I'd made Barbie and Ken kiss many times when I was younger (and hump each other). Why was it so much harder in real life?

There were aftershocks. When we returned to school the following Monday, I heard jeers and snickers while in the hallway venturing from class to class. Groups of girls and boys—some of whom didn't even know who I was—huddled together to gossip. A few made "kissing" noises at me.

It was equally as awkward passing Carter. I didn't know what to say or how to act. Was he going to try to kiss me again? Would I remember what to do? Or was I so bad at it that he was secretly contemplating how to dump me?

I couldn't take all of the heckling, which seemed to worsen every day. I decided that the only way to end all of the commotion was to break up with Carter. If we weren't together anymore, I figured, we'd be yesterday's news and the torture would stop.

My relationship with Carter ended almost as abruptly as it had begun. Time became my friend and the buzz about Carter and me quickly fizzled.

My friends' boasts continued to stick in my head, however. Their antics made my tongue tango seem like a game of tiddlywinks. They seemed so confident in their exploits. Would I ever become that comfortable? Would I grow into my vagina one day, or would it forever be labeled *Exit Only*?

SEVEN

Finger in the Pie

LUCKILY, MY VAGINA WAITED PATIENTLY IN THE WINGS FOR ME TO GET my shit together. I just needed a little more confidence, something that would gradually come with time.

Spring in Upstate New York: I was thirteen. The air was finally warming up and so were my hormones. I had yet another new boyfriend, a soccer player named Marcus. (Are you keeping tabs on the names of all of these guys?) We talked on the phone nearly every day—more than any other boyfriend I'd had before. I felt like I was in an actual relationship! Could this be the real thing? Only time would tell.

Marcus had short wavy hair that was somewhere between blond and brown. He never allowed a strand to be out of place. He was tall and thin, as most soccer players tend to be. The outline of his lips was curvy, almost lizard like; his devilish grin got me every time.

As I sat in Math class and dreamed of our future together, I would write my initials—replacing the F with a D for his last name (D'Angelo)—on the back of my notebook over and over again. Occasionally, the teacher, Ms. Wright, would shout at me to refocus my attention on the blackboard. It wasn't long before my eyes ventured back to my notebook. I had it bad for Marcus.

The bell rang for Math to end. I grabbed my notebook and pen, shot out of my chair, and hurried into the hallway. Marcus was already waiting for me with his back against my locker.

"Hey," he said.

"How was English?" I asked.

"We have another paper due next week."

"Oh," I sulked. "Do you think we can still hang out this weekend?"

"Yeah, Babe. Don't worry. I'll work on it on Sunday. My parents won't be home on Saturday. They're taking my sister to a tournament."

"Awesome! Can't wait."

He glanced around to make sure no teachers were in sight before planting a peck on my cheek. He had one more act to perform to fully demonstrate his adoration for me—taking a half-step back so he could slap my ass.

He's so dreamy!

"Call me tonight," I called to him as he headed toward his locker.

He spun around and walked backwards to reply, "I will."

"Boo!" my friend Tricia shouted at me from behind. She threw herself around my neck with a hug.

"Hey—are we still on for tomorrow?"

"Yeah," she answered. "Tell your mom to drop you off after lunch and then we'll walk over to Marcus's house. I told my mom we were going to Ishita's. She won't think twice about it."

"His parents definitely won't be home, so it's *on*."

We clutched each other's hands with excitement before running off to catch our respective buses home.

It's amazing how much things can change in only half a year. I went from dreading a French kiss to plotting out how to reach third base. I'd never been to a guy's house without his parents being home. This would be my first opportunity to be alone with a boyfriend for an extended period of time.

The next morning I woke up, jumped out of bed, and hurried to the shower. I wanted to be sure I was as fresh as a daisy for my intimate encounter. I selected my favorite button-down flannel tank top and a pair of tight jeans. I knew he was going to see my bra and underwear, so I made certain they matched.

Hours later, Tricia and I finally found ourselves at the doorstep of Marcus's house. We rang the doorbell and waited. We heard some rustling and thumping before the door inched open. It took a few seconds before a plump, brown-haired boy appeared in the doorway.

"Oh, hey Johnny," Tricia said.

"Hi, I'm Karin," I introduced myself as we entered the house.

I'd never met Johnny before since he went to a different school, but I figured he must be okay since he was friends with Tricia and Marcus. He seemed harmless enough.

"Nice place," Tricia admired, gazing up at the crystal chandelier.

I caught Marcus coming down the stairs and parroted, "Yeah, you have a nice place, Marcus."

As he descended the final steps and made his approach, I could see that he was wearing lacrosse shorts and a tee-shirt.

Understated. I like it—it looks good on him.

He planted a kiss on my lips.

Apparently, he isn't going to waste any time!

I kissed him back. Feeling all eyes upon me, I retreated backward.

Whoa, I need to ease into this situation. Find a way to stall the make-out session.

"Show me around," I insisted.

"Sure," he replied, continuing to play it cool.

He provided Tricia and me with a room-by-room tour of the house, explaining, as a thirteen-year-old boy would, the obvious purpose of each area. I feigned interest while pondering what we might do next—anything other than make out. By the time we entered his bedroom, Dustin—another soccer player from school—was already in there, immersed in a video game. I was relieved that there were so many people at his house. What's the worst that could happen with so many friends around?

"Super Mario Brothers—cool," I observed. "I'm pretty good at it. Can I play?"

"Sure."

I took the opportunity to plop on the bed next to Marcus's friend and grab a controller. We started playing.

Safe. The perfect distraction....

It didn't deter Marcus a single bit. He slid behind me on the bed and wrapped his arms and legs around me while I tried to beat Bowser and save the Princess. The instant my character ran out of lives and died, Marcus snatched the controller out of my hand. His hormones could wait no longer.

"Come on," he leered. "I want to show you something downstairs."

"Okay," I agreed, trailing him out of the room and down two flights of stairs.

"I have a workout area," he boasted, flicking on the light.

On reaching the bottom of the landing, I gaped at the expansive finished basement, which was filled with cutting-edge weightlifting equipment and free weights. "Wow, this is awesome," I raved, feeling a pang of jealousy. "You have so much space in this house."

"Check out the workout bench. Have you ever done bench presses before?"

"Me? No," I admitted.

"Here, let me show you."

He expertly raised and lowered the bar several times before replacing it on the rack. I gawked at his arm muscles. "See?"

"Yeah—you make it look so easy."

"I do it a lot. Here, sit down."

He sat up, patting the workout bench between his spread legs. I joined him sideways on the bench, so he was looking at my profile— as if this would provide me some sort of buffer.

His voice lowered as he said, "Don't be shy."

He shifted closer to me and grabbed my hand, leading it toward his shorts. The material of his lacrosse shorts left nothing to the imagination; he was already rock hard and bulging through. He leaned in closer and kissed my neck; it felt good, so I let him. He used his free hand to pull open his shorts and guide my hand inside.

"I don't know about this," I whispered.

"It's fine. Just wrap your fingers around me."

I can't believe it. I'm about to touch my first penis. I hope my hands aren't too sweaty. I don't want to gross him out or to give away how nervous I am.

I wrapped my hand around his penis.

It feels like a wrinkled, veiny, dry pickle. I'm so glad I didn't eat one with lunch.

"That's it," he reassured me, sliding his hands up my shirt and under the wire frame of my bra. We had reached second base before, so I wasn't bothered by his wandering hands. I tried to concentrate on what to do with his penis in my hand.

He sensed my hesitation. "Just move your hand up and down. That's all there is to it."

I began to jerk him off. It wasn't anything like what I had imagined. In my head, it had seemed like it would be a wildly passionate act. We would lie in front of a blazing fireplace on a bear skin rug, just like in the TV soap operas. But here, in the cool air of the basement, I felt bored and embarrassed.

How long do I have to do this? How do I know when he's had enough? My hand is already starting to cramp. I should have stretched it out first.

I stared at the wall as I continued to stroke him. Meanwhile, he kissed my neck and fondled my breasts.

Where's the magic? The fireworks? Maybe someone will come down and interrupt us, so this can end already?

We heard the basement door open and someone clopping down the steps.

My prayer has been answered!

In one gymnastic move, I rose, retracted my hand out of his shorts, and scooped my boobs back into their rightful cups.

Crestfallen, Marcus tucked away his little friend. "What do you want?" he snapped at our intruder.

"Can we ride your bike?" Johnny asked.

"Yeah, it's in the garage," Marcus relented.

"Come on, let's see what they're doing," I said, moving toward the stairs.

I turned around to make sure he was following behind me. He was there, all right, struggling to conceal his boner with a dejected expression on his face.

His friends awaited us at the basement doorway. They smirked at the sight of Marcus shielding his crotch with both hands.

"Go ride whatever bikes you want," he suggested. "Just make sure you shut the garage door."

"Don't worry," Johnny mumbled as the group scrambled toward the garage entrance.

Alone again. Damn it!

"Let's go to my parents' room," Marcus suggested.

Why would we go there?

I followed him blindly to his parents' bedroom, which was off the first-floor bathroom. There was no real privacy here, either. The wide bedroom windows overlooked the sloping backyard; anyone could have seen inside.

Marcus grabbed my hand and led me to the bed. "C'mere," he cajoled.

I had no control over what I was doing; I sat on the edge of the bed like a good girlfriend. My stomach started to ache. I had been so excited about this just a couple of hours earlier. Now that I was here, I felt like I was going to throw up.

I'm not nearly ready for third base. What's wrong with me?

"Lie down," he directed.

Nope. Not going to happen.

He eased my shoulder to coax me onto my back. He kissed me as I rolled over to face him.

All right, maybe this will be nice....

We made out for several minutes before he unbuttoned my shirt, exposing my bra. His eyes wandered down to the center of my jeans.

Crap. We both know where he's going next.

His hands raced down my waist to fiddle with the button and

zipper. I didn't help him, but I wasn't about to stop him, either. His hand slid into my pants. His long, thin fingers crawled closer to my vulva. My brain wandered far away....

His finger slipped into my vagina.

This is mortifying. I can't believe I'm letting someone do this to me. I'm not ready. Wait...do I hear a noise? What is that?

My head raised. I heard the sound even more clearly: snickering, from somewhere nearby.

"Do you hear that, Marcus?" I asked.

"I don't hear anything," he negated, kissing my neck. "Relax."

The noises turned into all-out laughter. I wrenched away from Marcus, but his finger was still tethered to my vagina.

"I heard laughing. I'm positive!"

"You're just nervous. No one's here."

Peering through one of the windows, I caught a glimpse of sneakers in motion.

I was right—they're spying on us! Pigs! This is over.

I closed my shirt and buttoned up my pants while retreating into his parents' bathroom. "I can't do this," I yelped before shutting the door.

I splashed some water on my face and washed my hands—as if they were the ones that required washing.

Marcus begged through the door, "I'll tell them to leave us alone."

"It's not that. I just don't feel good, okay?"

Marcus was respectful and didn't push the matter any further. I was grateful to him for that.

A few minutes later, everyone sat around the kitchen table eating a snack.

I wondered where my friend had been that whole time. Why hadn't she protected me?

"We better get going," I suggested to her. "We're supposed to be at Ishita's, anyway."

Tricia looked shocked. She didn't seem to understand why I was so anxious to leave. After eyeing me for another couple of seconds, she realized I was serious and conceded: "All right, if you say so."

"Wait—don't go," Marcus pleaded.

I could barely look him in the eye as I shot him down: "No, we have to leave."

Something changed. We'd moved too far, too fast. Just like that, our relationship had become tainted.

I gave him a quick obligatory kiss on the lips before shooting toward the front door. Tricia could barely keep up.

"Bye!" I shouted as we headed out.

Marcus pursued us and poked his head out the door. "Karin—call me when you get home."

"Okay," I agreed without turning to look back at him.

Once the front door closed and we were out of earshot, Tricia asked, "What happened back there?"

"I don't know. I felt really sick."

"I thought you liked him."

"I do...I did. I mean...I don't know anymore."

"Bummer, 'cause he's so rich. Your mom is going to be disappointed."

We walked for a few steps before Tricia cut to the chase: "So, what was it like?"

"What—jerking him off or having him finger me?"

"You did *both*?!"

"Yeah."

"Then *both*. I want to know about both."

I obligingly replayed all of the sordid details. She was mesmerized. I couldn't tell whether she admired me or was repulsed by me.

I couldn't wait for my mom to pick me up. I wanted to forget the whole day. This was nothing like what I had fantasized about; it most definitely couldn't have been anything close to love.

I knew having a boyfriend was only going to become more challenging as I grew older. Everyone's expectations would mature. I had to think things through better to avoid getting myself in another situation like this.

If this is what eighth grade boys want to do with me, what will they expect in ninth—blow jobs and anal?

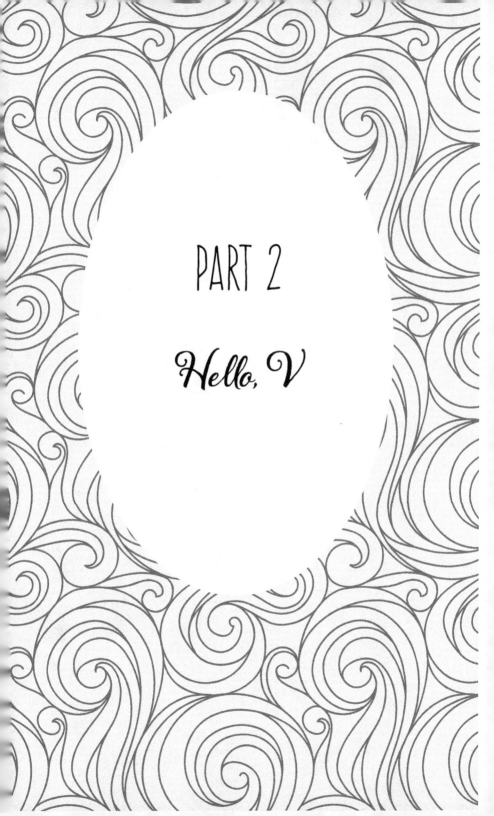

PART 2

Hello, V

$\mathcal{T}$he scene: Karin's bedroom, which is decorated in shades of white, mauve, and green.

Karin sits in the middle of her bed on a flowery bedspread, surrounded by throw pillows; she reads the latest issue of *Cosmopolitan*. She's dressed in an oversized tee-shirt and leggings with her hair in a high ponytail.

She hears an echo-like voice—like hers, but through a long tunnel.

V: *Psst…Karin.*
Karin: *(looking around, puzzled) Hello? Who's there?*
V: *Hey. Down here. It's me—your vagina.*
Karin: *Oh, hey vagina—I didn't know you could talk.*
V: *Call me V, we're going to be together for a long time. I can do a lot of things you don't know about. That's actually what I wanted to discuss. Can you put the Cosmo down for a second, please?*
Karin: *(setting the magazine on the bed) Okay, sure. What's up?*
V: *I'm not getting any younger in here. It's time to let me out of my box. Get me some fresh air. Hop on the saddle and take me for a ride, if you know what I mean.*
Karin: *Um, I hate to say it, V, but I don't know what you're talking about. Do you want a horseback ride or something?*
V: *Ugh, this is going to be a lot harder than I thought. (sighs) Girl, I'm*

ready for some action. Let me spell it out for you: A-C-T-I-O-N. Don't you see all the hot high school boys around you every day? I want to hump every single one of them.

Karin: Okay, settle down. I admit, I've totally noticed them, too. There are a few I really like. I can't decide who I should date. So many options—how can I choose just one?

V: Who said anything about dating?

Karin: Well, I can't just go around hooking up with random guys. I need to be dating them before we make out.

V: Really? Come on, girl, are we in the 1950s?

Karin: I don't want to be labeled as easy—or, worse yet, a slut.

V: By the time you land a steady boyfriend, I'll be covered in cobwebs. There's no better time than the present.

Karin: You listen to me, V. I'm the one in charge here. You'll do what I say.

V: Wanna bet?

Karin: You're just a vagina. (picking up the Cosmo) This discussion is over.

V: You have no idea what I'm capable of. Read my lips: We will have sex before the end of ninth grade.

Karin: (slaps the magazine down) No way—we can't have sex before marriage. My parents would kill me.

V: Who says they have to know?

Karin: If I get pregnant, they'll know. And God will know! I'm supposed to save myself for marriage.

V: Yeah, whatever. I usually spend most of the church service checking out the altar boys. Wouldn't you love to make out with Chris?

Karin: Yes, he is so hot. I've had a crush on him since third grade. But he told me I have a horrible voice in choir, so I'm pretty sure he's not into me.

V: Well, what about Brad? I've been eyeing him…Tony and Jerome, too.

Karin: They are to die for! I wonder if they think I'm pretty?

V: I'm sure they do. Why not get me alone with one of them?

Karin: *No! Stop it, V. (slamming her legs shut) We are not nearly ready to have sex. I should be at least sixteen! I didn't even like being fingered. Sex is probably worse.*

V: *Speak for yourself. I thought you'd never get to third base.*

Karin: *Ugh, are you sure you're my vagina? We don't seem to be on the same cycle at all.*

V: *Too bad. You can't get a new vagina. You're stuck with me, so we might as well learn to get along. Otherwise, I can make your life very difficult.*

Karin: *Are you threatening me?*

V: *Only if you rub me the wrong way.*

Karin: *Ha—what can you do to me?*

V: *Ever hear of the fifteen-day period?*

Karin: *That's not even a thing.*

V: *I told you I could do a lot of things you didn't know about. There are also pimples, sores…and don't even get me started on the yeast infections. You'll be able to bake enough Italian bread to feed the neighborhood!*

Karin: *You wouldn't…would you?*

V: *Don't fuck with me.*

Karin: *Look, V. I don't want any trouble. I just need a little time. This is a lot to process and things are very emotional for me right now.*

V: *Yeah, I guess you're right. But I don't want to wait too long for my first boning. It gets pretty lonely in here, if you know what I mean.*

Karin: *I guess it does. I didn't think of it that way…. We should start over, V. Let's be friends, okay?*

V: *You've got it. What should we do together first, girlfriend?*

Karin: *How about a hair mask in the shower?*

V: *Ooh, I'm in! Don't forget about the showerhead.*

Karin: *What do we need that for?*

V: *Don't worry, I'll talk you through it.*

Karin starts peeling off clothes as she dashes stage right toward the bathroom. Lights fade.

EIGHT

Bye, Bye Virginity

AH…THAT SPECIAL DAY WHEN THE BOY OF MY DREAMS (MY HUSBAND) *deflowers me. When will that day come? I know there will be a lit fireplace, a bear rug, candles, soft music, and glasses of wine. We will be madly in love and filled with passion, yet somehow resist temptation and take it slow…hours and hours of gentle kissing and caressing before the fateful moment when he would.…*

Okay, that's not at all what happened. I doubt many women lose their virginity in storybook fashion. This is how it actually played out.…

A few of my ninth-grade friends and I decided to attend a party at Brad's house. Why wouldn't we? This was *the* party house in town. There would be plenty of smoking, drinking, and laughs, as Brad's parents were known to be super cool.

While getting ready that afternoon, I didn't envision anything unusual or memorable was going to happen that night I wore a red Barbara Moss tee-shirt and jean shorts. (A girl never forgets what she wore the day her cherry was popped.) My hair was in its usual ponytail—which I made certain didn't have a single bump—and wrapped in a matching red ribbon tied in a bow. As I took a final look in the mirror, I experienced a wave of something exciting radiating from my body.

Is this what it means to feel sexy?

Upon entering Brad's house, a friend named Chris flashed an orange bottle of MD 20/20 (Mogen David wine, that is) from behind his back. "Want some?" he offered.

"Absolutely!" I replied, although this particular variety was far from my favorite. What right-minded girl my age was going to turn down free alcohol?

"Just don't let his mom or dad see it, okay?" he warned as he filled my cup.

"Yeah, no problem," I shrugged. I was playing it cool, but I had more important things on my mind. "Um…do you know where Brad went?"

I hadn't seen the host yet, and I was dying for a glimpse of his dirty blond hair and devilish smile.

"Yeah, he's out back by the pool. Did you bring a suit?" he asked.

Before I could respond *No*, he was already off pouring MD 20/20 for another girl. I laughed to myself as I made my way through the sliding doors to his backyard and headed up a hill.

It was a steamy summer evening in Upstate NY. The warm breeze felt great on my skin as I made it to the landing where his trampoline and pool were located. Brad was perched atop the slide, about to make his descent. His eyes locked with mine before my eyes wandered to his bare chest.

He's so cute….

Since I didn't have a suit, I ogled him from the edge of the pool. Occasionally, he swam over and splashed me. I relished every minute of attention from him. Brad was a hot commodity around school. Every girl liked him—even the ones who were a grade or two older.

How can I possibly compete against them? What would he see in me? I have a mouth full of braces and, being Italian, I'm cursed with having upper lip hair. Not exactly the recipe for a beauty queen.

Despite all of my glaring flaws, Brad exited the pool, wrapped a towel around his waist, and approached me.

"Want a cigarette?" he asked shaking the water out of his hair.

I wasn't about to turn down the offer, even if it was one of those shitty Camel cigarettes he always smoked. I was a Marlboro Light girl myself. "Sure, thanks," I accepted.

Naturally, he didn't have any on him, since he'd just exited the pool. "They're in my room," he invited. "Come on."

He was halfway down the hill before I could get my feet to move. I scurried to catch up with him so no one could cut in between us. We broke through the middle of the party and made our way up the stairs to his bedroom without any interference.

Brad ushered me in and closed the door, which had a hole in the center. I surmised that something had pissed him off, causing him to punch it or pummel it with an object, such as a baseball bat. He stuffed a white sock in the hole to avoid prying eyes. Naive kid that I was, I didn't think anything of it.

His bedroom was lit with a black light—a trendy thing back then.

As promised, he offered me a Camel cigarette and positioned an ashtray for us. We lit up, made small talk, and reminisced. Before I knew it, the cigarettes were extinguished in the ashtray and we were lying down on his bed making out.

He is a really good kisser….

Things progressed. I allowed his hands to wander around my body. It must have been my awesome cigarette breath that excited him enough to ask, "Have you ever had sex before?"

"No—"

"Do you want to?"

One would think I'd need some time to process such a major question before giving a thoughtful response….

"Yeah, sure," I blurted.

Whoa—what am I saying? Did I just agree to having sex?

"You go, girl!" V cheered.

"Oh no, not you again."

"This is perfect—he's hot and experienced! I can't think of a better person for us to lose our virginity to."

"I can't believe we're even considering having sex," I argued. *"I'm*

way too young. Aren't I supposed to wait until marriage?"

"You can wait for marriage all you want. In the meantime, I'm letting his snake in the garden!"

"Fine," I conceded to my vagina. "But we do it on my terms."

"Do you have a condom?" I asked Brad.

"Of course," he answered, displaying one in his hand.

"Wow!" V marveled. "He's a magic man!"

I climbed on top of Brad, my eyes locked on his as I slid his penis inside of me. It was a little uncomfortable, but the first time is supposed to hurt, right?

"Hey," V called. "I hate to disturb you, but something very wrong is going on here."

"Quiet, V. I'm concentrating. I know it's going to hurt a bit, but—"

"Hurt?"

"Sshhh!"

"All right," V sighed. "You'll find out soon enough, I guess."

Ignoring V, I eased up and down on his penis, my teeth glowing like white Chiclets in the black light. After what felt like ten minutes but was probably more like two, Brad slid his hands around my butt. His facial expression went from blissful to shock.

Am I bad at this? Am I doing something wrong? Does it hurt him as much as it hurts me?

"You've got it in the wrong hole!" he yelped.

Shit, shit, shit. I'm such an idiot. How did I screw this up?

"Don't say I wasn't trying to warn you," V scoffed.

"Keep your trap shut!" I shouted at her.

Thank God the black light was on, so Brad couldn't see my embarrassment. I slipped off him, terrified.

It was clear that Brad needed to take control, which he did. He flipped me on my back, fumbled around a bit, and hit the jackpot: He was finally inside me. The real hole, that is.

"Whoo-hoo—now you got it!" V exclaimed.

I ignored her, staring at the ceiling.

How could I not know the difference between my anus and my vagina?

How come no one prepared me for this moment? I don't remember covering it in Health class, and my mom certainly never discussed it with me.

Brad continued to pump away, but I was far removed from the moment. I was unaware of whether he finished or not, but I suspect he did. Either way, it was over before I knew it.

He helped me find my clothes and then dressed himself. I wanted to bask in the moment, but I dreaded what he might share with others.

Meandering through the house in a daze, I rejoined the party with him downstairs. This marked my first "walk of shame," although it certainly would not be my last. I was met by stares from the other girls and smiles and winks from the guys. I should have anticipated this. Everyone knew what went on when Brad brought a girl to his room and closed the door.

I ducked into the nearest bathroom to regroup. I had to pee anyway, given the drinks in my system.

I was mortified by what was in the toilet bowl, on my underwear, and even on my shirt and shorts.

Oh no! Did I get my period?!

There was no way I could hide so much evidence.

I was startled by a knock on the bathroom door.

"Just a sec," I responded.

"It's Brad. Are you okay? Open the door."

"I'm okay. Give me a minute."

I wiped, flushed, and washed my hands in a desperate attempt to pull myself together. I opened the door a crack and poked my head out.

"There's blood all over me and the bed," he whispered. "Are you all right?"

"Yeah, I think so," I said, opening the door a bit wider so he could see my dilemma. "It's all over my clothes, too."

"Stay here. I'll get you something."

He disappeared. I closed the door to hide out for a few more minutes.

Brad returned with a sweatshirt that was long enough to cover over the spots on my shorts. At that moment, he was my knight in shining armor. I was so relieved that he was being cool about everything, which was his nature.

No one at the party believed that I was cold; it was a warm summer evening, and the house didn't have air conditioning. But walking around in blood-stained clothes was not a good look.

Later on, my dad seemed to buy my cold story when he picked me up. I was silent during the fifteen-minute ride home through dimly lit back roads that further helped conceal any errant stains. I couldn't help but wonder if he somehow knew what I had done. When we arrived at my house, he asked me to open the manually operated garage door, as he always did. The car's headlights stared me down like I was a convict making a jailbreak. I was sure he was going to notice something off about me.

I hope he doesn't see this blood. What if he has a sixth sense and already knows what I did? I gotta get out of here.

Before he could have a chance to say anything, I ran through the garage to the side door, shot inside through the kitchen, and made my way straight to my bedroom. The sooner I could get out of these clothes and into my pajamas, the better.

In the privacy of my room, the evening's activities replayed in my head.

I did it. I finally had sex.

"You mean WE, don't you?" V asked.

"Yeah, I guess. But I blew it...I mean, anal sex? Really?"

"Don't sweat it, girl," V countered. *"You skipped ahead a few steps."*

"V...can I ask you something?"

"Sure...as long as it's not about the mishap. I wouldn't go around telling anyone about that, if I were you."

"I agree one hundred percent...what I need to know is...did we do it right?"

"What do you mean?"

"I mean, is that all there is to it? I don't feel any different. I don't get

what the big deal is. It wasn't great; it wasn't bad. It just was."

"Listen closely. I'll tell you what the big deal is: the orgasm."

"Orgasm? What's that?"

"Oh, you'll know when you have one. It will be the most amazing, body-quaking pleasure we'll ever experience."

"That definitely didn't happen tonight," I confessed.

"Well, if at first you don't succeed, try try again."

NINE

The Cat's Out of the Bag

As it turned out, the first time I had sex also became my first one-night stand. Go big or go home, right?

Brad would always have a special place in my heart, and we remained good friends—but nothing more. Neither of us ever brought up our intimate evening; we acted as if it had never happened. Oddly, I was fine with it. I was relieved to have rid myself of the daunting task of losing my virginity. Best of all, my parents never found out. And, now that I'd had sex, it didn't seem like such a bad thing; in fact, V and I were very much interested in trying it again.

By sophomore year, my sexuality was in full bloom. I fell for a hottie named Carson, who was a junior. He had short dark hair, brown eyes, and a slender build. The taller and skinnier the boy, the more I seemed to like him. He was smart but, like me, didn't apply himself. He played hockey, which I found really attractive because it was my favorite sport. (My dad would take me to Binghamton Whalers games when he got tickets from NYSEG, the company he worked for.) I enjoyed attending Carson's games and watching him play. There was something very appealing about a man in uniform checking another guy on skates.

It didn't take long for us to establish that we were seeing each other, which essentially meant I had a steady boyfriend. But I made him wait two full weeks before getting it on. Since he was a year older, I wasn't sure how long I could keep him hanging. The truth was, I wanted it just as much as he did.

There was something special about my sexual encounters with Carson. For starters, I didn't make the same mistakes I did with Brad. The best part was that our make-out sessions lasted a really long time. Thinking back, I'm not sure how he managed to hold off so long. Maybe all of the weed in his system made it take longer for him to get off. I'll never know.

Wednesdays were my free day—no dance and no cheerleading—so I always went to his house after school. His mom worked late, which gave us plenty of freedom. To be on the safe side, Carson would slide a knife into the molding around his bedroom door to jam it shut, just in case his mother came home early.

"What do you want to listen to?" Carson asked, moving toward his stereo system.

"How about The Beatles again?"

"Sounds good," he said, taking the *Abbey Road* CD—our go-to album—out of its case and placing it in the six-disc changer.

I threw myself down on his waterbed and floated on my back for a moment as the water rolled and then settled. I looked over at a large tie-dyed tapestry hanging on his wall and then at a poster of Bob Marley on his closet door that stared back at me.

Carson crawled on my body, sending another wave of motion through the bed. He leaned in for a kiss. The anticipation was already building up inside me. We both knew where this was leading.

He took his time, undressing me as we kissed. He wrestled a bit with my button fly jeans before I leant a helping hand. He remained calm and cool throughout and neither of us uttered a word. There was no need to talk; we just listened to the music and experienced each other.

My eyes were shut ninety-five percent of the time, so it felt like night. The other five percent, I peeked through my eyelashes to check if he was looking at me. Occasionally, I met with his sweet brown eyes staring at me. I panicked and squeezed mine closed. My mind tricked itself into thinking that, if my eyes were closed, he couldn't see me anymore.

Carson genuinely enjoyed foreplay. He didn't sprint to the finish line. He sucked on my neck for what felt like an eternity, leaving a regular pattern of hickeys on my skin. He gently flipped me over on my back to manually stimulate me. We kissed deeper as his slender fingers worked their magic.

How did I get so lucky? It's like he knows exactly what I want him to do.

Three or four songs into the album, we found ourselves ready for the main event. He slid on a condom ever so carefully. I didn't care to watch; there was something about it that felt like a private moment between a man and his penis. When he was done, I would give it a once-over to be sure it was on properly before allowing him to penetrate me. (Not that I had a clue back then about how it should look once secured.) I trusted him but, at the same time, was well aware of what a horny teenage boy might try to do.

He took command, displaying his rough side. He flipped me over doggystyle and went to town. His bony hips pressed up against my backside over and over again.

I feel like I need to let him know he's doing a good job. But how?

In some movies I'd seen, people made noise when they made love.

I don't even know how to make those sounds. What if I sound like a dying seal or a cat giving birth, instead of a hot, moist girl? I have to at least try…here goes nothing.

I began to make some subtle sounds—deep breaths, a few moans, an *ugh* here and there. The harder he went, the more sound I released. He seemed pleased by my performance.

Eventually, Carson could hold out no longer and ejaculated. But he didn't just roll over and light up a cigarette. He sheltered me in his arms with my head on his chest, as we floated on the waterbed. I felt loved.

Everyone was happy, right? Nope—not V.

"Psst...hey, down here...sorry to interrupt. I know you're baskin' in the moment and floatin' on a cloud or whatever...but I'm pretty sure there's more to this sex thing. A LOT more. What about the Big O I've been tryin' to tell you about?"

I ignored her, satisfied with Carson's attentiveness.

The days passed. I turned up the volume on my sex sounds. Turns out, I was good at this pretend passion; however, the more I faked it, the less I began to enjoy the act of sex. My partner thought he was the shit, as most high school boys do, so he convinced himself that he made me come every time. Who can blame him? I sounded like a porn star, ready to drench the sheets like a firehose.

Then, one Friday afternoon, we had a little conversation....

Carson's older brother had picked us up from school and brought us back to their house. We were both starving, so we decided to order in subs and peach Snapple, which was my favorite flavor. His mom had left a twenty-dollar bill on the counter for us. The delivery would take at least a half hour.

Back then, when we were fifteen, hungry, and didn't have food, only one solution came to mind: cigarettes. With that in mind, Carson and I made our way out to the back deck, which had a screened in porch. I reached into my back pocket for a fresh pack of Parliament (P-Funks, as we referred to them). They seemed cool to us because they had the recessed filter. I ripped off the cellophane wrapper, removed a cigarette, and shoved the pack into the front pocket of my jeans. Carson was ready with the lighter as I put the cigarette between my lips. It was windy, so he made a cup with his other hand to help it light.

"Thanks," I said. "Oh, did you see Mr. King's face today when I was late for Science? I thought he was going to send me to the office."

"Yeah, you're lucky he didn't. You were, like, one away from lunch detention. He's such a prick," Carson stated, exhaling smoke from his own cigarette.

"I know," I agreed. "He hasn't liked me since seventh grade. I don't know what the hell I ever did to him."

"Who knows. He probably just needs to get laid."

"Yeah, me too," I joked, grabbing him by the belt buckle for a kiss. I released him and continued, "Right after the food gets here. I'm freaking starving!"

"I'll give you something to eat," he remarked, grabbing his junk.

"Don't tempt me," I flirted back.

"Speaking of sex," he continued, taking another puff. "Seemed like you were really into it yesterday."

"Yeah—I mean, it was good."

"Good? You were moaning and breathing pretty heavy. Must have been some orgasm!"

The words hit me like a ton of bricks.

Orgasm? What orgasm? He seriously thinks I had an orgasm? I don't think I've ever had one of those. How would I even know if I did?

I took a drag of my cigarette while I contemplated a response.

Should I be truthful?

I'd read an article in *Cosmo* about faking orgasms. Had I unknowingly been doing this with Carson?

Is our entire relationship based on a lie? What a bad girlfriend I've been.

My stomach twisted into knots; I was overcome with guilt. Not to mention that fact that I wanted to have a genuine orgasm and longed for the first one to be with him.

Maybe, if he learns the truth, he'll try a little harder? Yeah, that might do the trick!

"Um, hello. Earth to Karin—it's me, V. Somehow, I get the feeling that isn't exactly the best approach."

I dismissed V's warning, instead blurting to Carson: "Well, I've never had an orgasm, ya know?"

I could tell by his dropped facial expression that I'd wounded him. *Badly.* But once it was said, there was nothing I could do to retract the words. There was no walking them back.

"What do you mean you've *never had an orgasm*? What about all the noise you make?" he demanded.

He looked like a puppy that just got put up for adoption. His brown eyes winced as he took the last drag of his cigarette and extinguished it in a metal ashtray.

I tried to explain: "Well, it feels good, so I make noise...but...I haven't ever actually come."

Ouch.

I had no idea this would be such a blow to his ego. It was as if I'd criticized his penis size. I suppose, however, if the tables had been turned and I found out that he'd never gotten off during sex, I would have felt the same—maybe even worse. My mind raced to figure out a way to ease his pain.

"I haven't had an orgasm with *anyone* before," I explained. "It's not *you*, it's *me*."

I hoped that might help reassure him, but it didn't. He was well aware that I'd only had sex with one other person, which wasn't much of a sample size; the stats were not in his favor.

I wish he was high right now, so he could forget we were having this conversation.

The doorbell rang: delivery.

Phew! Saved. Dinner has arrived.

Eating in front of the TV was a welcome distraction for both of us. We became engrossed in an *X-Files* rerun and attempted to solve the latest mystery. Carson didn't act like himself. For the most part, he remained silent in a chair on the opposite side of the living room. I suppose he needed time to process what I'd said. I tried to remain upbeat and keep the conversation going, but it was futile.

After dinner, I fully expected we'd head off to his room and lock ourselves in with the knife in the door, as always. For the first time ever in our relationship, he declined to have sex.

What? No sex? On a Friday night! This is bad—very bad. I'm too young for this shit.

Five long days passed before we resumed normalcy. From then on, I was under massive duress to achieve orgasm. I could barely focus on what we were doing. I kept hoping *today would be the day*. It felt like it was right around the corner.

The longer I went without an orgasm, the more frustrated I became and the more I took to faking it. Sitting alone in my room one evening, it became clear to me I needed some advice about how to get to the next level—but whom could I ask?

Oh, I know! Why didn't I think of this sooner? "Hey, V. Are you there?"

"I'm not on an all-inclusive vacation to the Bahamas—so yeah, I'm here. Spit it out—what's the problem?"

"About this orgasm thing.... The other day, Carson and I were having sex. The second he finished and pulled out, I felt like I was seeing stars—it was euphoric even."

"I remember—that was a good one! Your man delivered the goods!"

"So, was that it? Did I have the Big O?"

"How the hell should I know? I've never had one, either."

"But...I thought.... You were making it like you're the expert: the all-knowing vagina."

"Like you, I'm a pretty good actress. Fake it 'til you make it."

"Fuckin' hell, V, you suck! I need real advice here, or I'm going to be forty and orgasmless."

"That's not even a word. What're you so worried about, anyway? You and me, we're enjoying the game of hide the salami with that scrawny love machine."

"Yeah, we are," I considered. "But my friends keep talking about the Big O. I want to experience what they feel. Natasha said it was absolutely amazing—the best thing she's ever felt. When's it my turn?"

"Girlfriend—don't get so worked up or it won't happen. Lay back, relax, and enjoy. Our day will come."

V was full of shit, but I held onto a little glimmer of hope.

One day, my body is going to explode in ecstasy. My quest for the Big O is on and nothing will stop me.

TEN

Cysterly Love

AT LONG LAST, ALL WAS FORGIVEN, AND CARSON AND I RESUMED our journey to Orgasmville in his adult-free house. Marlena and her boyfriend, Ken—who had joined us for the car ride in Carson's new Jetta—were looking forward to finding Orgasmville together, too.

We pulled into the driveway and hopped out with our backpacks in tow. Carson snuck us inside through the garage door.

The four of us climbed up to the top level where the bedrooms were located and parted ways as couples: Marlena and Ken headed to Carson's mom's room; Carson and I ventured into his. I always felt bad when people had sex in his mom's bed, but I kept my mouth shut, not wishing to ruin anyone's good time.

"We only have an hour," I reminded everyone. "We can't be late to cheer practice or coach will make us do extra jumps."

"Got it," Ken acknowledged.

I admit to having been a little jealous. Marlena was a frequent visitor to Orgasmville. She and Ken usually only needed about five minutes for a satisfying round trip excursion.

I followed Carson into his room. I tried to think optimistically, but I had my doubts.

Maybe this time will be different…I hope.

"*You and me both,*" V chimed in.

"Sssh, *you keep quiet*," I snapped.

He closed the door behind us. While he worked on jamming his knife in the door, I tossed away my bookbag, unzipped my windbreaker, and flung my sneakers in the corner of the room before hopping on his bed.

"*Don't forget to give him the coaching you learned*," V called to me.

It occurred to me that she was right: I did have a useful pointer to share.

"Okay, Martina told me that you must determine the exact location of my G-spot," I offered, realizing after the fact that I probably sounded like my Health teacher.

He shot me a blank stare. Having two older brothers, you'd think he would have at least heard something about the G-spot. "Where's that?"

"In my vagina," I replied.

"Yeah, no shit. But *where* in your vagina?"

"*Jeez*," V remarked. "*This guy needs to listen to Dr. Ruth on the radio.*"

"Deep inside it," I said, ignoring V. "Way in the back, I think. You just gotta get your dick as deep as you can."

"Well, I like the sound of that," he grinned.

His expression sent a warm rush through my body.

"*All right,*" V reflected. "*Something's happening...all systems operational!*"

He pulled my shirt over my head. We knew we had limited time, so the bra stayed put. I struggled to get his belt undone and shimmied his pants down to his knees before calling upon a foot to help pull them down the rest of the way. His boxers—the ones I had bought him for Christmas—came down right behind them. It was clear he didn't need any time to warm up; his soldier stood at perfect attention.

"Condom?" I questioned.

"I got one."

While he fumbled around in his dresser drawer, I used the free moment to remove my own pants and hot pink underwear.

He found a condom, tore it open, and rolled it on. There was nothing holding us back from hunting for my G-spot. Away we went. He started on top. It felt good, but the same as always. He couldn't manage to get in any deeper than he usually did. I looked up at him and shook my head *no*. He knew it wasn't doing the trick, so I suggested straddling him.

Since I remained a smidge self-conscious, I didn't sit upright. Instead, I leaned forward, so our bodies were pretty close with only about four inches separating us. It felt like he was getting in a little deeper. I rode away until my legs started to tire.

Ten minutes passed before he checked in: "So, you almost there?"

"Almost where?"

"Ya know, orgasm?"

"Right now? Um...I don't think so. How do I know if it's the G-spot or not?"

"I know what we should do," he decided, rolling me onto all fours.

He grabbed me by the hips and set up behind me. He thrust his hips back as if to give his penis a running start. He plunged in as deeply as he could with all his might.

"*Ow!*" I howled.

"*Ow!*" V reiterated.

The upper half of my body collapsed on the bed as a shooting pain raced through my entire vaginal area. The shockwave radiated to my stomach.

"I'm sorry. Are you okay?" he asked, completely frozen.

"No," I answered. "That really hurt."

"Do you want me to stop?"

Yes, please stop.

V was in total agreement: *"I'm waving the red flag. Something's really wrong on the battlefield. That soldier of his needs to retreat!"*

"No," I answered. "Just go a little easier."

"You're kidding me. What's the matter with you?" V asked.

I ignored V as he gently reinserted himself and resumed thrusting.

Despite his care, the pain didn't stop; if anything, it grew in intensity.

I bit my lip and took one for the team. I couldn't let Carson or V down.

After a while, Carson could tell we were getting nowhere and that I had stopped being an active participant. He satisfied himself right away, so he could put me out of my misery. As soon as he pulled out, my body slumped to the bed in a fetal position. I closed my eyes, absorbing the unbearable pain. Water pooled in my eyes.

"What have we done to you, V? I'm so sorry."

She remained silent—down for the count.

"Can you grab my underwear?" I peeped.

"Yeah," he said, scrambling to find them under the covers. He fished them out and tossed them over to me.

"You need to put them on me. I can't move."

"What's wrong?" he asked, providing assistance. "Did I go too hard?"

"I don't know. This seems like something else. I've never felt this type of pain before."

"Oh man, I hope it's not your appendix or something."

"Don't even say that...but you might be right. Can you get me some Tylenol or something?"

"Yeah," he responded.

He dressed himself, left the room, and returned right away with the pain reliever.

I raised my head just high enough to pop two Tylenols. Carson proceeded to help me complete getting dressed—one limp limb at a time. Meanwhile, in the other room....

"Oh my God! That's it, right there! Do it! I'm coming! I'm coming!"

This was a clear-cut case of insult to injury: Marlena was floating around Orgasmville. By this point, she'd earned a role as the town's tour guide.

Carson consoled me, stroking my hair while we waited for my agony to subside.

A few minutes later, Marlena and Ken—radiant and fully dressed—entered the bedroom through the open door.

"We made your mom's bed," Marlena announced.

"Whoa, what happened?" Ken reacted.

"Are you all right?" Marlena followed.

"I don't know," Carson replied. "All of a sudden she felt a ton of pain."

"Aw, what's the matter? Carson's dick too big for ya?" Ken joked.

Carson picked up the nearest object he could reach and chucked it at Ken's head. I appreciated that he had rallied to my defense but was too incapacitated to celebrate.

Marlena knelt down next to me. "Are you able to walk?"

"I haven't tried yet."

"Come on, Carson, help me get her up."

They each grabbed an arm and propped me on my feet, while Ken retrieved my bookbag. The pair walked me down two flights of stairs and back to the car. Every time my foot hit the floor it felt like a knife was stabbing me from my uterus through to my anus.

The ride back to the high school was utter hell. The slightest bump caused my insides to feel like they were going to explode. We finally reached the school, where the group helped me out of the car.

Carson and Ken weren't allowed to come in with us, so we said our goodbyes.

"I wish I could make you feel better," Carson said, kissing me.

"I know you do. I'll call you when I get home from practice."

He nodded with his puppy dog face before heading back into the car. I leaned into Marlena as we hobbled through the front door.

"How am I going to cheer?" I asked.

Of course, it was a rhetorical question. I was in no condition to do any physical activity, much less cheer.

"We'll tell the coach that you're sick. You have a really bad stomachache."

At least there was some truth to this. My stomach definitely hurt.

The coach took one look at me and approached with a stern look on her face. She looked this way even when she smiled.

"What's wrong with her?" she asked Marlena, as if it were her fault.

"I have a stomachache," I chimed in. "I can barely walk. It started about a half hour ago."

"Right. Well, sit down for warm-ups and then we'll see how you feel in a bit."

Marlena ushered me to the nearest wall. I put my back up against it and slid my back down just before my tush was about to hit the ground. I put my hands out to gingerly lower myself.

Ouch! Even this hurts.

The other girls warmed up: They ran laps, practiced arm positions, did planks, worked their abs, and performed jumps.

I thought I might pass out. I needed fresh air. The gym was stuffy and the noise made me feel even worse. I attempted to rise, hoping no one would notice while I snuck off to the bathroom.

Suddenly, a hand grabbed my arm. It was the coach.

"Come on, I'll take you," she offered. "I don't want you passing out and falling on my watch."

"Thanks," I said.

I entered a bathroom stall and sat on the toilet. I waited for something—anything—to happen that might alleviate the pain. In the midst of stage fright, I had a hard time getting my body to pee. I felt the urge to poop, but there was no way that was going to happen with the coach in the room.

"How's it going in there? Feeling any better?"

"Not really. I can't do anything. It just hurts."

"We should call your parents to come get you, then. No sense having you suffer on the floor all night."

Music to my ears!

All I wanted to do was curl up in bed.

But what will I tell my parents? Certainly not the truth....

"Have you ever had an ovarian cyst before?" the coach asked.

"I don't think so. What's that?"

"It's a fluid-filled sac in or around your ovary. They can rupture from time to time and cause severe pain."

"Do you think that's what this is? It's really awful," I winced.

"Might be. Especially if you've been having sex."

Sex! Who said anything about sex? How does the coach know I had sex?

"Well, I'm a virgin, so it can't be that," I lied.

"Hmn," the coach considered. "Maybe it's a cyst, maybe not. Either way, you should go to the doctor first thing tomorrow."

"Okay," I blurted.

I flushed and washed up before the coach escorted me to the pay phone. I avoided all eye contact with her, just in case she might suspect something. She pulled a quarter out of her pocket and dialed the numbers I fed to her.

My dad arrived within ten minutes. The coach helped me into the car and handed my belongings to him. I sprawled my body across the back seat of our Dodge Intrepid for the grueling ride home.

I spent the evening lying down on our couch opposite the TV.

"What the hell's wrong with you?" Debra prodded. You look like crap!"

"Yeah, no shit, Sherlock. I feel like I'm dying."

Debra started out of the room when I switched my tone and urged her back: "Hold on. I have to pee, but I can't make it to the bathroom. I need your help."

"What? Help you pee? Help you to the bathroom? I can't carry you."

"Come on, just try," I pleaded. "Forget it. Just get me something I can use to prop myself up. Every step is like a dagger tearing into me."

"I got it!" she shouted, bounding up the stairs.

Great. Where is she going? I really need to pee.

Debra reappeared a couple of minutes later holding a pair of Rollerblades.

"Rollerblades! What am I supposed to do with those?"

"Trust me."

She placed the Rollerblades on my feet and laced them up. When she was done, she yanked me off the couch. I teetered in pain as she shifted behind me. "Here—I'm going to give you a push to the bathroom."

Well, I'll be damned. This sounds stupid, but it just might work.

She gave my back a shove and I was on my way. Sure enough, I rolled into the bathroom without unnecessary additional pain. It worked so well, in fact, that I wore the Rollerblades everywhere in the house and Debra pushed me from room to room.

I ended up seeing the gynecologist (unfortunately, a male), who confirmed the coach's cyst diagnosis. I thought for sure he'd prescribe something for the pain, but no. There was nothing for me to do except take over-the-counter pain reliever, as needed. And, girl, did I need it!

For the next two days, I popped the pills while Debra continued pushing me around the house. It worked well for the most part, except when she occasionally pushed too hard and I'd fly into something. To this day, I'm not sure whether these mishaps were accidental or on purpose. Overall, though, she was immensely helpful to me, which was a big deal considering how much we usually argued and fought. Perhaps this was her way of showing me cysterly love— something I would always appreciate.

ELEVEN

Roast Beef Lips

By senior year, my relationship with Carson fizzled out. We never did officially make it to Orgasmville. Despite all of our efforts, it just wasn't in the cards.

A few other partners came and went. Nothing crazy, I wasn't boasting double digits or anything like that. My confidence was growing, and I became less ashamed of my body than in previous years. That said, I still had a lot to learn about love and sex.

Interestingly enough, my next lesson would not come from a boyfriend. Instead, Bryce—a good friend who played hockey with Carson—gave me an education I would never forget. He was two years older than me but was still living at home while he attended a local community college.

It was a wintry Saturday afternoon. Since I had my own car, a red Geo Prizm, I was able to venture out in the snowstorm and didn't need to rely on my parents to cart me around. I picked up Martina and headed over to Bryce's house, where we holed up in his basement, along with three high school guy friends. We cracked open our first twelve-pack of Beast—otherwise known as Milwaukee's Best—and mindlessly stared at the TV.

Bryce flicked channels. Nothing seemed to appeal to him or the group—until he came up with an idea: "Hey, wanna watch a porn?"

Porn? I've never seen one of those before! Should I act disgusted? On the other hand, this sounds kind of intriguing....

My parents didn't have anything resembling porn lying around the house. The most perverse thing I'd ever seen was a toothbrush with boobs that my dad kept in his top drawer. And I certainly was never going to risk getting caught going behind the curtain in the darkened adult section of the video store.

This could be my only chance....

"Hell yeah!" I shouted.

I was often seen as one of the guys, so no one blinked about my enthusiasm. Before I knew it, a dozen VHS tapes were strewn across the floor.

"Which one do you want to watch?" Vincent asked me.

I examined the covers one by one.

Which one to choose? There are so many—I had no idea there could be so much variety!

I recall one tape with a heavily made-up blonde woman on the cover—not that anyone would be looking at her hair. Her breasts were gigantic: *Guinness Book of Records* size.

How does she stand up straight with those boobs? They must weigh at least ten pounds...each!

The cover of another one showcased a teasing, less busty brunette in a checkered schoolgirl skirt. Her legs were invitingly spread apart, exposing her white underwear.

This is such a tough decision....

"What do you want?" Bryce urged. "Big boobs? Big cocks? Threesomes?"

How should I know? Hmn.... Which one would earn a thumbs-up from Roger Ebert? I hope the acting is good.

My deliberations were taking too long. Vincent randomly picked up a tape and tossed it to Bryce, who inserted it in the machine.

I laid on the carpet on my belly, propped my chin up with my hands, and prepared to watch the action.

I didn't have long to wait. This film didn't bother with exposition, character development, or plot; it cut the formalities and headed straight to penetration. Close up.

A vagina was right there, on the screen. A well-hung male pumped in and out.

Who on earth would allow herself to be taped having sex like that? I'd never have enough confidence to do such a thing.

"I don't know…never say never," V said. "*Someday I might like the spotlight.*"

"*The only spotlight you're getting is the one at the gynecologist's office.*"

As shocked as I was by what I was viewing, I could also feel myself getting aroused. My skin became flushed and warm to the touch. There was no mistaking it—V was fired up!

We stared in silent stupefaction until Bryce yelled out, "Check out that roast beef!"

The guys chuckled. "Yeah, her lips look like some dried-out roast beef, all right!" Vincent remarked.

Roast beef? Is that what they call it? Do I have roast beef lips?

I began to feel self-conscious. I wanted to run to the bathroom and find out. If I looked like deli meat down there, I vowed to never again have sex with the lights on.

The vagina in the subsequent scene was cute, pink, and much softer-looking than the previous one.

Man, I hope mine looks more like this vagina….

I felt like I was wearing see-through pants and everyone was trying to determine if my vagina was like this one or more resembled a slab of old, dried-out roast beef. I began to feel overwhelmed and needed a break. I rose to my feet.

"Where are you goin'?" Vincent asked. "Too much for ya?"

I tried to act tough and maintain my bad girl reputation: "Just goin' for a quick smoke. Anyone wanna join?"

No one budged.

"I'll be back," I announced, turning toward the stairs.

"My parents won't be home until late. You can just smoke down here. But don't get any ashes on the carpet," Bryce warned.

Damn it. I'm stuck.

"Are you sure?" I asked.

"Yeah—wouldn't want you to miss the money shot."

The money shot? What could that be?

I didn't want to look too puzzled, so I just smiled and pulled out a cigarette. Bryce handed me an ashtray. I allowed the lighter and smoking logistics to distract me from the movie for as long as possible, then reclaimed my spot on the carpet.

A few minutes later, I learned the definition of a "money shot."

The goo—what seemed like a pint of it—went all over the woman's face and hair. The guys laughed appreciatively, while I tried to remain cool. V was just as repulsed. She dried up like—dare I say it, roast beef!

That is gross. I will never allow a guy to do something like that to me.

The rest of the evening was anticlimactic, as it were, and I drove back home in the snow to make it in time for dinner. I washed my hands and joined my family around the table.

"Did you have fun at Bryce's?" my sister asked.

"Yeah, we just hung out and watched TV."

"Sounds real educational," my dad remarked sarcastically.

Ha! If only he knew....

My mom chose that exact moment to enter the room with a steaming dinner tray.

Oh no...it can't be! What are the odds?

"Roast beef," my dad salivated, waving his knife and fork. "Delicious."

This must be some bad cosmic joke. I'm pretty sure the universe is punishing me for having watched porn.

I stared at the roast beef on my plate: Sure enough, it was overcooked with dark brown edges.

"Who would like to say grace?" my mom prompted.

My sister volunteered and everyone dug right in—except me. My hands, which grasped my knife and fork, were paralyzed over my plate. I just couldn't unsee the dried-out roast beef vagina from the porn flick. It leapt from the screen right onto my dinner table. The resemblance was so uncanny I had to smother it with mashed potatoes. Unfortunately, this made it worse, conjuring images of the money shot in my head.

Later that evening in the bathroom, when my head had a chance to clear, I grabbed a hand mirror and checked V out up close.

The moment of truth. Here we go, V. Don't let me down.

I hesitated for a moment as I slid the mirror between my legs. Of course, all I could see was black curly pubic hair. I used my fingers to gently part the dense shrubbery that protected V. Clearly, the Brazilian wax concept hadn't made its way to suburbia yet. My eyes widened as I took a closer look.

Well…what the hell is this?

It didn't resemble roast beef—but it wasn't that light pinkish color, either. This wasn't in the video. Maybe that particular vagina wore makeup? Or is mine an anomaly? Someone needs to publish a vagina manual—with color photography, of course.

"I like to think of it as 'coral,'" V chimed in. "Kind of like those roses you wore in your corsage for junior prom. It really brings out the best in my clit."

"If you say so, V. I can live with it, as long as I don't become the poster girl for an Arby's ad."

TWELVE

Karin Does Myrtle Beach

THE DATE: SPRING BREAK, 1998.

The place: The Budget Inn, Myrtle Beach, South Carolina.

The scenario: Six girls in one hotel room; a half-dozen guys in the other. The rooms are joined together by a shared balcony.

We had the perfect recipe for an epic spring break. We started drinking early, went all day, and continued through the evening and into the next morning. We had keg parties with funnels, went to the Freaky Tiki and danced on tables, and, as I now admit, got laid. A *lot.*

I know, it probably sounds like I had become a slut—especially on the heels of having just described watching my first porn video and characterizing the color of my vagina—but at least my spring break sexcapade was all with the same guy. I prefer to think of this as a carefree, innocent time. V and I were young and free-spirited, just enjoying single life and all of the pleasures it had to offer. Why not? We had zero responsibilities (or parents) for the entire week.

During one of my few restful moments during spring break, I decided to sun myself with a couple of other girlfriends on the balcony while simultaneously allowing my freshly painted nails to dry. I wore my new purple bikini with the "boy short" bottoms, which were all the rage that year. I'd overheard the guys talking that morning about some former high school grads showing up and staying at the hotel across the street. I didn't pay much attention to it—until one specific name caught my attention.

"Yo, Brian!" Mario called from our balcony toward the hotel across the street.

My ears perked up. I just *had* to get up and peek over the railing. I was pretty sure the particular Brian being summoned was considered one of the most gorgeous guys from our high school.

Could it really be him?

"V—*wake up. You're gonna want to see this.*"

I took one look at his well-toned, slender body, tanned skin, perfectly styled brown hair, and chiseled jaw and confirmed that he was the Brian of my dreams. Every girl had the hots for him, and I was no exception.

I can say that I knew Brian, but he didn't know me. I'd watched him grace the halls of our school with his dreaminess on countless occasions, but we'd never spoken to each other. I became determined from that first sighting to correct this oversight and catch his attention.

"Hurry up, man!" Brad yelled down at Brian, who stood beside his car with an overnight bag flung over his shoulder.

To answer your obvious question: *Yes*, this is the same Brad who had taken my virginity. And *No*, we never made any mention of the anal thing, or the mess caused by our brief encounter.

Brad continued, "We got a keg tapped up here, so come on up once you're checked in!"

"Be right there!" Brian shouted back.

My pulse raced in anticipation of his arrival. A couple of minutes passed before I heard a few raps on the balcony door. I didn't want to seem too eager, so I held my position sunning myself. I gave a subtle glance his way, just to let him know I was aware of his presence.

Brian acknowledged my friends and me with a flick of his wrist— the smoothest Brad Pitt-like greeting possible. "Ladies," he said with a twinkle in his eye.

I tipped my white-rimmed sunglasses down to get an even better look and followed with "Hi." I hoped I hadn't overplayed my interest; I wanted to leave just enough room for him to wonder.

He sauntered across the balcony into the guys' room to fill up a plastic cup with beer. Two friends followed close behind him.

My eyes followed him the entire way.

"*Damn, girl,*" V addressed me. "*I'm feeling a little moist down here. That's the dude for us! I'd like us to—*"

"I know, I know, *you don't have to say it!*"

From that point on, I wore the skimpiest outfits possible and ramped up my flirtations. By the second day, May—one of my friends—took notice. "Karin, what are you doing?"

"What do you mean?" I smirked.

"You know exactly what I mean—with Brian."

"I don't know," I pretended. "I guess I'm just having some fun."

"Well, yeah, but ya know…."

Her widened eyes were trying to tell me something. I had no idea what it was.

Is she trying to give me a warning?

I shrugged, which caused her to unleash an "Ugh" intended to let me know just how thick I was. "I think he goes both ways," May revealed.

"What?" I gasped.

"I heard he's *gay.* He's always wrestling around with guys…and there are rumors about him."

"Stop it! He *is not.* A guy that hot can't be gay," I insisted.

The more I thought about it, though, the more plausible it seemed. Maybe he was *too* sharp, stylish, and well-groomed. "What a waste," I sulked.

I couldn't completely let go, still needing some kind of verification one way or the other. I brought it up with anyone who would listen, hoping someone would confirm it was just a rumor.

Later that evening, I was still no closer to an answer. While we were sitting and drinking on the balcony, Brian called me out: "Hey,

Karin, I hear you're telling everyone you think I'm gay."

Shit. Now he thinks I'm the one who has been spreading the rumor!

My cheeks flushed red as my mind raced for a response. I could feel everyone's eyes penetrating me.

Ah, I've got it!

"Prove me wrong," I teased in the sexiest voice I could conjure. My face drew closer to his.

Without missing a beat, his hand slid around to the back of my head. His fingers became lost in my long hair as he pulled me against his lips. Before I knew what was happening, his tongue was dancing in my mouth.

Wow, he is good at this! There is no way he is gay.

"Whoo-hoo!" V reaffirmed. *"Time to celebrate!"*

He tastes so good, like a beer-flavored mint—if such a thing even exists.

"Damn!" Mario shouted. "Get a room."

Realizing we had taken center stage, we reluctantly peeled ourselves apart. "Touché," I remarked.

There was nothing more for me to say. I had my answer and now desperately needed a cigarette—because, yeah, the kiss was *that good.*

Realizing I had left my Parliaments behind so no one would swipe them, I slinked across the balcony into my adjacent room where May was doing her hair. I made a heart with my hands and mimed it beating out of my chest.

She looked bewildered so I explained, "He just kissed me."

I shot her a wink while grabbing my secret stash of cigarettes and then sprinted back to the balcony. There was no way I was about to let anyone else cut in on my lover boy. He was all mine.

Whatever had transpired between Brian and me was not over—not by a long shot. The sexual tension between us continued to build as the evening went on. I lost count of how many drinks I'd consumed throughout the day or anything else that had happened up until the moment the two of us were passionately engaged in the guys' filthy bathroom. The real world—including the raucous party right outside the door—ceased to exist. Time stood still.

"You're beautiful, you know that?" he complimented.

Part of me was aware that he was feeding me a line to seduce me, but I didn't care. It was all part of the game, and there was no time to waste. I couldn't resist his looks, his charm, or his six-pack. He had become something of an unattainable prize. I'd snagged someone I considered out of my league.

We wanted each other with an equal amount of lust. He couldn't remove my shorts and underwear fast enough. He didn't protest when I asked him to put on a condom which, of course, he had at the ready.

We went at it like maniacs, starting on the toilet lid, moving to the shower (which was off), and ending up on the sink. He placed me on the edge of the porcelain facing him and went to work. Every thrust sent chills down my spine. I let my fingers wander across his chest feeling his rock-hard pecs and then down to his washboard stomach. Electricity shot through me as Brian kissed my neck and shoulders. I didn't ever want the moment to end.

We were ill-prepared for what happened next. Something wet was squirting all over my back. I barely had time to think about it before we heard a crack. My butt began to slide off the edge of the sink as I fell backwards. Brian, meanwhile, was too caught up in the moment and in no hurry to disengage. He used his superhuman strength to keep his penis firmly in place, while V held on to his member for dear life. I continued to tumble down, yelping as he pulled me in tight. Thankfully, his efforts prevented me from striking the floor.

Although I was only ninety-seven pounds, my weight had apparently been enough to detach the sink from the metal pipe that ran up from the floor.

"What do we do?" I panicked.

"Move back to the toilet," he suggested.

"*Sounds like a plan!*" V advised.

"*Yeah, this is mind-blowing. Hands down the best sex we've ever had. I can't spoil it now. The sink can wait. I really think he can get us to the Big O!*"

We shifted over to the toilet without missing a beat. At some point we became aware that Chris, a mutual friend, was pounding on the door and screaming, "Will you two get out—I gotta piss!" A moment later he added, "What the fuck are you doing in there? Why is there water coming under the bathroom door?"

Um, maybe this is a sign?

Brian got the picture and rushed to complete his business. I enjoyed the encounter, but the interruption caused yet another fail in my quest to reach the Big O.

We pulled ourselves together, draping on our soggy clothes as best as we could. We tried to shut off the pouring water, to no avail. We sheepishly exited the bathroom to find a room full of stares. Despite the flood, some people cheered and applauded. Others sneered in disgust.

While I retreated back to my room—partly victorious, but mostly in shame—Brian and a couple of guys called the front desk and dealt with the bathroom disaster. I didn't have any plan except to lie down on my bed and try to recover from what had just happened. Unfortunately, a nasty surprise awaited me: My lovely friends had moved all of my stuff to the couch and decorated my pillow and blanket with an array of colorful condom packets.

"We booted you to the slut couch," Martina cackled.

Why am I a slut for doing what comes naturally? Brian will probably get high-fives and become a legend for the accomplishment. Meanwhile, I'm slut-shamed.

I don't recall if I cried or not, but I wanted to.

I hoped everything would settle down, but this was not the case. The female security guard, whom we affectionately dubbed Patch because of the black patch over her left eye, appeared on our balcony.

Oh no, now I'm really in trouble.

She was there to break up our party, while a stocky maintenance man with a comb-over appeared beside her, presumably to fix the broken sink.

Everyone else had shifted out of the two hotel rooms and crammed shoulder to shoulder on the balcony. Like magnets, Brian and I ended up next to each other. "There they are," someone shouted from within the crowd.

How humiliating. How will I explain this to my parents?

"You're on your own from here on out," V said.

"Thanks. Why do you always disappear at the first sign of trouble?"

I turned to make a break for it when Brian reached out to prevent me from moving.

"I'll take care of this," he reassured me.

Clearly, he had some sort of plan. He turned his attention over to Patch, wrapping his arm around her and guiding her into the boys' room. I might have been jealous if she were hot and fifteen years younger, but this wasn't the case. I was just hoping he could sweet-talk us out of whatever trouble we were in.

A few minutes later, Patch emerged from the room with a plastic cup full of beer and a cheerful expression on her face. She remained for another hour, mingling with the balcony crowd and every so often refilling her cup. So much for breaking up the party!

Whatever Brian had said to Patch did the trick and got us off the hook. No one ever asked me to pay for damages. I marveled at his talent for bullshit.

The party resumed, during which I clung to Brian. With his help and several refills of beer, I started to feel better about the day's events. A couple of hours later, things started to wind down and it was time for bed.

Once everyone dispersed, I found myself back in my room with the girls, where things had returned to normal. We changed, went through our beauty routines, hit the lights, and tucked ourselves in. Although my friends had eased up on the taunts, I decided to own my place on the slut couch and sleep there for the night.

It was pitch-black and eerily silent. I took a deep breath, hoping I could fall asleep as visions of Brian's six-pack filled my mind. Then, through the darkness, Jessica's voice peeped out: "So...what was he like?"

An outpour of laughter followed, lifting my spirit. Instead of feeling embarrassed, I wanted to spill the details—every last one. "He was fucking amazing!"

"I totally would have banged him in that bathroom, too," Martina admitted.

I proceeded to give the girls a play-by-play, and all was forgiven. If anything, they seemed to admire me.

Brian and I were inseparable for the remainder of spring break. The following afternoon, I snuck across the street to his hotel room in the hope we might avoid any interruptions. It was a lot easier for him to kick two guys out than for me to displace five girls.

We picked up right where we had left off: round two of earthshaking, mind-blowing sex. He took his time, savoring every moment as he celebrated my body like no other guy had before. He licked and kissed every inch of my skin from head to toe. He drove me wild while spending plenty of time on my inner thighs. I kept thinking the Big O was imminent. If he couldn't make me orgasm, then no one could. Unfortunately, despite all of his noble efforts, it just didn't happen.

"What's wrong with us, V? Why can't we get off?"

"I don't know," she replied. "I think you need to go back to the drawing board."

"What do you mean?"

"Cosmo, Elle, Seventeen. One of those magazines might have the answer. If not, it won't be a waste of time—I like how I feel when you read those articles."

"All right. I guess it couldn't hurt."

Whenever I had the opportunity, I gathered up women's magazines and resumed my research. Sure enough, while flipping through a *Cosmo*, I hit upon a letter from a reader who asked the billion-dollar question: "Why can't I orgasm during penetration?"

I held the magazine inches from my face, absorbing every word of the response and uttering the vital bits aloud: "'Clitoral stimulation. Eighty percent of women can't orgasm from intercourse alone. Focus on the clitoris.'"

"Oh my gosh, V, that's it! I'm not screwed up! These guys don't focus on the clit!"

"There's hope for us yet!" V cheered.

At last, we had our answer. Brian may have set the bar pretty high, but there was still room for one man to claim top spot. All he needed to do—whomever he ended up being—was play me like a Super Nintendo game controller. Surely, I thought, there is one guy out there who is up for the challenge. How difficult could it be? A Super Nintendo controller has four buttons: A, B, X, and Y. Easy peasy—I only have one clit.

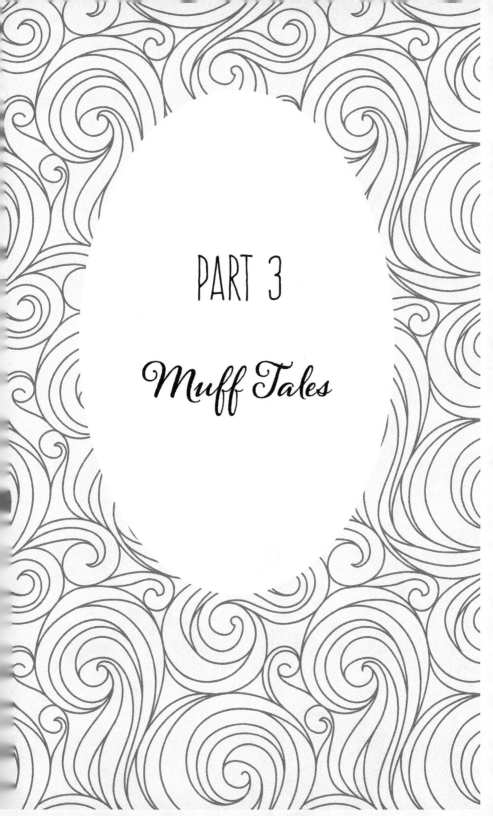

PART 3

Muff Tales

even.

Is it really a lucky number? I can't really say, except that it was meaningful for me. You see, by the time I left for college, I had been with a total of seven guys. Was that too many? Too few? Or just right?

I had no idea how to begin to answer any of the above questions. One thing I did know was that I wanted a fresh start when I stepped foot on the SUNY Brockport campus. While I longed to be popular and continued to be a partier, I also wanted to be a good girl and have a clean reputation. In other words: Have fun without being labeled a slut.

Was this paradox impossible to achieve? Seeing as I was a Dance major, most of my time would be spent in the dance studio anyway—not exactly a hotbed of guys. I figured I'd at least give it the old college try.

As usual, V had a mind of her own. Little did I realize that it was filled with other plans.

THIRTEEN

Frat Boy Lust

ONE OF THE MAJOR REASONS I CHOSE SUNY BROCKPORT, BESIDES for the Dance program, was for the Greek life. I had always wanted to be in a sorority—mainly because where there are sororities, there are also fraternities!

By the second semester of my freshman year, I was well initiated, as it were, into the Sammy circle. "Sammies" was a nickname for members of Sigma Alpha Mu fraternity. Come formal time—which is like a prom for college students—it seemed only natural to be invited by one of the brothers, Tim—as friends, of course.

Fortunately, I had brought all of my high school prom gowns to college. By the end of freshman year, I was rocking some serious freshman fifteen, which put me at about 115 pounds. To say I was partying a lot would be a major understatement; if drinking had been an Olympic sport, I could have made the team and been their captain. It was a miracle I still fit in my senior prom dress.

I was pledging Alpha Sigma Alpha (ASA) sorority. My pledge name was Zienna, but a bunch of the sisters took to calling me Z. (Though no one else was aware of this, V appreciated that we were now V and Z.) My pledge sisters and I primped in our dorm as we geared up for a long night of dancing and drinking.

"Raelie—remember that guy I was telling you about?" I asked

a sister while applying another layer of mascara to ensure my eyes would stand out. "The cute one whose hat isn't quite backwards but isn't really to the side, either?"

"Yeah," she casually replied. "I meant to tell you, he's pledging Sammy."

How could you forget to tell me such important information?

I flipped out: "Oh my God, he'll be there tonight!"

I had seen Backwards Hat Boy—as I referred to him, because I didn't know his name—around campus a few times. He worked at the dining hall, usually at the ice cream station. A few months earlier, I had asked him for a dish of mint chocolate chip with hot chocolate sauce. He was so nervous that he knocked all of the cups into the sauce container. I laughed, but thought he was really cute as he struggled to stand the cups back up and hand the ice cream to me.

Now was my chance to get to know him better and find out if he shared my interest. I was only going with Tim as friends, so I figured there wouldn't be any harm in ditching my date at the right time without hurting his feelings or embarrassing him.

"The pledges are the DDs [designated drivers], so he won't be drinking...but he'll be there," Raelie informed me, adding: "I'm not wearing any underwear tonight."

"Wait, what?"

No underwear?

"*If I could get a word in here,*" V intervened. "*I, for one, would love to free-buff! I could use the fresh air!*"

"No way," I replied to V. "*Not happening.*"

Still, I continued to weigh my options.

It could provide easy access for Backwards Hat Boy....

What, is he so lazy he can't push my underwear aside?

But...I'm in college—why not throw caution to the wind?

No. I don't think I can walk around with my chocha uncovered. My dress is pretty loose from the bust down...underwear is a necessity. It makes me feel safe...from what I don't know. Pathogens in the air? Bacteria on seats? Something getting stuck on my pubic hair? Stray dicks?

What if I get my period? Or my body just decides to secrete vaginal discharge? That's why women wear underwear!

"Yeah, cool, good idea," I lied polishing off the last sip of my vodka cranberry.

I had no intention of going anywhere without wearing underwear, but I didn't want to seem prudish to my friend.

Soon we were dressed to the nines and it was time to leave. I was greeted by Backwards Hat Boy the moment I approached the front steps of the frat house. He ushered us onto the bus with Lars, another pledge. I'd met Lars over the summer, so I took the opportunity when I was walking past him to lean in and ask the name of my dream boy.

"Oh...him—that's Damien. But you can call him Deylah," Lars grinned, either because he was high or because he knew I was into his friend.

"Thanks," I said as my date dragged me up the bus stairs. I couldn't help but longingly look back at Damien, wishing he would accompany me to the formal instead.

The bus drove us to Hickory Ridge Country Club. It was only supposed to be a fourteen-minute drive, but it seemed a lot further at the time. Maybe it was the alcohol?

Tim, my date, was kind of short in stature, not particularly fit, and had a tendency to talk out of one side of his mouth. To make matters worse he was rolling on ecstasy—which wasn't my scene. He kept asking me to massage him, so I separated from him shortly after we arrived at the banquet hall.

The party rocked into gear, but Deylah was nowhere in sight. The DJ played my kind of music: hip-hop. It didn't take long for me to become officially hammered, dancing like I was in a music video while scanning the room to see if Deylah had arrived. By 11:00 PM, I was drenched with sweat from nonstop dancercise.

Out of the corner of my eye, I spotted the pledges arriving to pick up some of the brothers and bring them back to Brockport. Deylah was among them. His baby face, dark brown hair, and slender build attracted me right away. His clothes were oversized for his frame, but that was his style—even while dressed up in khakis and a button-down. His trademark Detroit hat was positioned in its normal fashion atop his head.

I had no control over myself; the alcohol took over. Next thing I knew, I found myself walking across the dance floor as if I were in a tunnel, heading toward the light: him.

I went straight up to him and laid it all on the table. "Do you want to come home with me tonight?"

Maybe I'm coming off a tad forward?

"Yeah," he muttered.

His reserved and mysterious demeanor made me yearn for him even more.

"Okay. See ya later," I waved, returning to the dance floor.

"Where are you going? The bus is this way," he gestured. "That's why I'm here, to bring everyone back." He peered around nervously. "First, I just need to ask Brother Tim if I can actually go home with you."

"Why? He's not going to care. We aren't dating."

"That doesn't matter. I'm a pledge. I can't just take a brother's date home without getting permission first."

"What's he going to do—paddle you?"

Tim chose that precise moment to creep up from behind and swing his arm around my shoulder. "You're not trying to steal my date, are you, pledge?" he asked Deylah.

Oh, shit. This is not going to end well.

"Well, actually Karin asked me if I would go home with her, so…."

"Oh cool, well, whatever," he stammered. "She doesn't roll anyway."

I'm right here, dude. I can hear you.

"Thanks, brother," Deylah said, shaking Tim's hand.

I was amazed by how easily Tim had let me go. No argument, no tussle, nothing. I was insulted and pissed for a fleeting moment about not being worth fighting for, but then realized how ridiculous that was, since I'd gotten exactly what I wanted.

I was distracted from my thoughts when several sorority sisters headed out of the banquet hall.

"Come on, Z!" Raelie shouted.

I followed in earnest, making sure I stuck close to my frat boy. I plopped myself in the seat beside him. He shyly looked out the window while we waited for everyone to board.

During my freshman year, I had a real thing for Jolly Ranchers and made sure to always have some candy on me. I pulled a packet out of my purse and plopped a grape one in my mouth.

Now's a good time to kiss this hot frat boy!

I leaned over and drunkenly whispered, "Do you like Jolly Ranchers?"

"Yeah, why?"

My mouth lurched towards his. My tongue rolled the Jolly Rancher into his mouth. Everything went dark, except for the brightly colored stars that danced behind my eyelids.

We're kissing! Success!

It seemed like forever until we returned to my dorm room. We had the place all to ourselves. I put in a DMB (Dave Matthews Band) CD and slipped into my sexy jammies.

Oh yeah, they were sexy alright—plaid flannel pajama pants and gray Vestal High School Football '98 tee-shirt. What a turn on for my frat boy!

"What are you thinking?" V pressed. *"You literally have zero sex appeal right now. You're going to blow it for both of us."*

"Relax, I got this," I replied to her.

One might think prancing around in my bra and underwear would have been a better option, but I was wearing my mom's old strapless bra from, yep, you guessed it—JCPenney. It was pretty ratty and my boobs were too small for it, so the cups were slightly indented.

While lighting a candle, I caught a glimpse of myself in the mirror.

Dear God, I look like a ghost!

My skin was pale white, and my mascara had run under one of my eyes. A few bobby pins had come loose from dancing and were sticking out of my hair. I attempted to wipe off the mascara while making a dash for the light switch. The room turned pitch black, except for the candlelight flickering from my desk—and not a moment too soon before my frat boy could see me up close in the light.

I hopped up to the top bunk. It was pretty easy for me to get up there given my size and familiarity with the angles. Then it was Deylah's turn. I found it amusing watching him scale the side of the bed and try to avoid bumping his head on the ceiling.

We made small talk, but it didn't take long before we were making out. He still tasted like the grape Jolly Rancher I had transferred to him on the bus.

I could lie here and kiss him forever. This is heavenly.

My stomach filled with butterflies as his large hands lured me closer. I loved the feeling of being completely enveloped by him. He used his tongue to explore the upper half of my body. I was amazed by how much of my breast fit in his mouth.

"*Why don't you send him down my way!*" V exclaimed.

I had no doubt of this. She was dripping wet with passion. We both wanted to screw him so badly, but I remembered my challenge to wait.

V is saying "Yes," but my head is telling me "No."

The old expression goes that "guys only think with their dicks." Well, I admit I was in the same predicament; I was allowing V to do the thinking for me. I toyed with the idea of just letting him have it.

What's the harm? He has a condom.

My hand roamed into his pants. My fingers were met with something unexpected—a warm, sticky blob.

Crap—he's more moist down there than I am!

Amidst all of our foreplay and our humping, he'd had a premature ejaculation. I didn't know whether to be annoyed or flattered. I went with the latter.

Damn, I'm good!

Unquestionably, he was one satisfied customer. We snuggled up and fell asleep in each other's arms. There was no room for either of us to move; if we had, someone would have ended up on the floor.

Someday, Deylah was going to become special. At the time, I had no clue just how special. I could reveal this to you now…but nah. I don't want to be premature myself.

FOURTEEN

Sacked

HELL WEEK.

And yes, it was a literal hell for me. Not only was the pledging process exhausting, I wasn't permitted to have contact with anyone except sorority members. This meant Deylah and I were off-limits to each other.

Finally, one Saturday morning, it was over. I became an official member of ASA. My pledge sisters and I couldn't wait to celebrate… right after we took a nice long nap, a necessity after having been sleep-deprived for seven days.

I hadn't been in my dorm room for over a week. I had forgotten to bring my medication, Procardia, with me while I was away, which was pretty dumb. I had been diagnosed with Raynaud's disease—an autoimmune condition that results in poor blood circulation. The beta blocker was intended to help promote better circulation. On my arrival in the dorm room, I went straight for the prescription vial, which was on my desk mixed in with a bunch of pens and highlighters. I swallowed one pill down with the remains of a water bottle.

What a relief.

There was only one *little* problem. The red label on the side of the bottle clearly said, **"Do Not Drink Alcohol."** Well, I was a college freshman—a newly indoctrinated sorority sister, no less—so going on the wagon was not an option. Caution had already sailed away in the wind.

Then V presented me with a devastating surprise: my period!

"Oh, come on. Now?"

After I cleaned up my feminine nightmare, I spent a couple of hours rejuvenating before joining some friends at a local bar, where we used fake IDs to get in.

I would have preferred to spend time with Deylah but, as luck would have it, he was next to go through hell week. It seemed unlikely that we were going to pick up where we had left off anytime soon.

At the bar, I ordered my typical bottle of Labatt Blue and socialized. I flitted from group to group—proudly wearing my letters—talking to sisters and friends from classes. Occasionally, when a good song came on, I'd let loose on the dance floor.

While I was on my way to a much-needed bathroom break, one of the older sisters tapped me on the shoulder from behind.

I spun around to face Dreyae, a sister with dark black hair and a sharp jawline. For a second, I thought she was going to yell at me. Instead, she shouted over the music, "Someone wants to meet you!"

"Me? Okay, sure," I agreed, peering around to identify the guy. "I don't see anyone. Who is it?"

"One of the football players. He said he's been watching you all night and thinks you're really cute," she teased, finally cracking a smile.

A football player? Shut up! I've never been asked out by a football player before.

I tried to stay calm, even though I felt anxious—so much, in fact, that I skipped the bathroom break. "Cool, take me to him."

She grabbed my hand and led me to the far end of the bar. A sea of football players parted and, in the middle, stood a handsome guy with dirty blond hair and pecs bursting out from under his tight shirt. He cracked a half-smile as he set his beer down on the bar to shake my hand. "Hi, I'm Christian," he introduced.

"*V likey!*" V said.

"*Me too, V. Me too.*"

"Karin—but everyone calls me Z."

Before I knew it, Dreyae had left me to fend for myself. Fortunately, Christian and I hit it off instantly. Although the blasting music made it difficult for us to hear each other, our body language conveyed more than enough. After several drinks, I'd forgotten about Deylah.

Last call. I had a moment of panic that I might lose Christian, but he didn't waste a second inviting me back to his friend's house.

As we floated through the streets together, he complimented, "You look amazing."

"Stop, you're just saying that," I blushed.

"No, really. You're super hot."

I was hooked.

We marched hand in hand to his friend's house, where I was pleased to find that a regulation-sized beer pong table had been set up. Plastic cups, ping-pong balls, and ample amounts of beer were positioned and at the ready.

This is my game!

I was eager to impress Christian. We won match after match and ran the table. I lost count of our victories and beer consumption after a half dozen of each. My brain swirled and my eyesight became blurry from the mix of alcohol and medication.

It must have been after three in the morning when I found myself locking arms and strolling with Christian across campus. I was smitten, to say the least, but nearing blackout phase.

V took over the controls as I began to fade in and out of consciousness.

Next thing I knew—perhaps an hour later—I found myself topless in his bed, kissing him sloppily. His pecs pressed against my breasts.

Damn, he has a good body.

"Oh, hey, you're finally awake," V noticed. "You've been missing all of the action."

"I see you wasted no time getting down to business," I said.

"He's a fine specimen if I've ever seen one," she marveled.

Uh oh. Fading fast....

I couldn't keep my eyes open. I felt the room dancing around me. Another blackout. I'd left my fate entirely up to Christian...and V.

◉ ◉ ◉

Several hours later. My head felt like it was in a vice. I didn't dare try to move. I became vaguely aware that I was exposed except for my underwear and part of a rumpled sheet. Tiny bits of sunlight flashed through my lashes but, try as I might, I couldn't open my eyes.

"Morning," an unfamiliar voice said.

Where am I? Who is that?

"V, what happened last night?"

Nothing. She was down for the count.

Besieged by panic, I finally mustered enough strength to open my eyes. I looked up at a scraggly stranger in a loose jersey who stared at me up close. "Looks like you and Christian had quite the night," he smirked.

"Who are you?"

"Nick—his roommate."

I felt obliged to be polite and return the introduction: "Karin... call me Z. Where's Christian?"

"Ha!" Nick laughed. "He's lying right next to you."

I rolled over to face the equally nude football hunk. He was wide-awake and chipper. "Hey there, Sleeping Beauty."

Now I know you are full of shit. I am anything but a beauty right now.

I desperately tried to piece together what had transpired the night before. Given our current state, I worried we'd consummated. I prayed he'd used a condom if we had. The last thing I needed was to get pregnant or contract a venereal disease.

I pondered how I might delicately ask him for some details about the night before, at least to calm down my fears. Then another one hit me....

Oh, shit! My period. I couldn't have had sex. My tampon must be overloaded. What if he saw it when he went down on me?

"I'm going out for bagels," Nick offered. "Any takers?"

"Yeah, I'll have a sesame with cream cheese," Christian replied.

"No, thanks," I declined, although I really did want one. I desperately needed answers to at least one of my questions and wanted Nick to disappear.

The moment he headed out, I fell out of the bed and rummaged around for my clothes. Fortunately, everything was there, and I managed to get dressed.

I scooped up the rest of my possessions and searched through the bedding for telltale signs of my period. I could not have withstood the humiliation if I'd left bloodstains on his sheets. For all I knew, it was like a Freddy Krueger bloodbath in there.

"What are you looking for?" he asked.

"Nothing...nothing," I answered in relief. Everything appeared to be clean.

I stumbled toward the door.

"Where are you going? Why such a hurry?" he asked.

"I have dance rehearsal at 9:00 AM," I lied, unable to look him in the eye.

"I'll call you later," I bleated, exiting his dorm room.

I couldn't return to my dorm fast enough. Along the way, I fumed at V.

"You've really done it this time, V. You've gone too far!"

"Me? I'm not the one who blacked out. Maybe you should stop drinking so much."

"It wasn't the alcohol, it was that damn medicine...."

"Well, sorry," V said. *"You missed a damn good time, girl! Wish I could provide details."*

On arrival at my dorm, I went straight to the bathroom to change my tampon. Only…it wasn't there. Gone!

What could possibly have happened to it? Did I take it out while in the throes of passion? If so, where did I put it? Did I politely go to the bathroom and flush it—or did I do something trashy, like whipping it out in front of him? Is it lying in a garbage can in his room?

The unanswered questions mounted. The torment was more than I could bear. In an effort to wash away the night, I took a steaming hot shower, inserted a new tampon, and returned to my room. Determined to make sure this would never happen again, I tossed the prescription bottle in the garbage. If I had to make a trade-off, there was no contest; drinking would win every time.

Later that day, Christian called and asked if we could get together on Friday. I hesitantly agreed. I had reservations only because I was mortified at what might have occurred. Then again, how bad could it have been if he was asking me out?

For a moment, Deylah popped into my head. I kept picturing his baby face and felt guilty about my wild night with Christian. There was no reason for me to feel bad—it wasn't as if we were in a relationship—and yet, inexplicably, I did.

I shook it off and turned my attention back to Christian. When Friday arrived, we made plans to meet up at the bar. My period was finally over, but I had no intention of engaging in sex. For the foreseeable future, V would have to take a back seat. It was my only attempt at retaining some level of dignity and not being perceived as a jock groupie.

This time, after drinks and laughs at the bar, I made certain to bring Christian back to my room. I felt I could control things better in my own domain.

As we rolled around in my bed and his hands traveled down my body, I whispered, "I'm really sorry, but I can't. I have my period."

Yes, it was a lie—but a good one for two potential reasons. First, it would prevent us from going further than I wanted. Second, if he were to say something along the lines of "Well, that didn't stop you the other night," I'd know we went all the way.

But he didn't. He seemed content restricting the action to just the waist up.

I was pleased with myself on a few fronts: I'd ditched my medication; managed my alcohol intake; and kept V in check. I nestled my head in a comfortable spot on his chest as we drifted off to slumberland.

@ @ @

I woke up early the next morning coherent, but with a different issue than the prior morning after: Christian's massive arm was crushing my upper body. I wiggled my way out of our entanglement and climbed down my bunk bed ladder.

I felt good about myself—and about Christian. He had respected me the night before and it didn't seem as if there were any repercussions from the night I'd blacked out. I stepped out of my room into the common area to stretch my legs when I noticed my roommate Carla seated on the community couch.

"Hey, what are you doing out here?" I asked her.

"I didn't want to interrupt when I saw you had a visitor," Carla answered.

"You could have come in. We weren't doing anything."

"Next time you better lock the door though, cuz Deylah was just here. He saw you with Muscle Man and ran out with a real pissed off look on his face."

"No!" I shrieked. "Are you kidding me?"

"It all happened so fast," she admitted. "I saw him when he came in. He asked me if you were in there. I didn't know what to say and froze. Before I could respond, he was going through our door."

Fuckin' Carla! Ruining my life.

I grabbed my head with both hands and hunched over in shame.

He hasn't forgotten about me, after all. His hell week was far worse than mine. He probably didn't have any way to communicate with me. *What have I done? How could I not have waited just a few days for him? I've really fucked things up.*

Wracked with guilt, I retreated to my room and politely kicked Christian out.

Oddly, he obliged without asking any questions. He kissed me before departing. I half-heartedly kissed him back.

I'd only briefly known Deylah, but at that moment I was certain of my feelings for him. I devised a plan to make things right.

After showering and completing my other bathroom rituals, I rummaged through my closet for a baby pink crop top and my shortest pair of white shorts. I blow-dried my hair and tied it into two high pigtails, securing them with pink heart-shaped ponytail holders. I applied a generous amount of makeup and the darkest pink lipstick I had in my caboodle. I checked myself out in the mirror.

"*If you don't win him back looking like this, it's hopeless,*" V assured me.

"*Thanks. This isn't going to be easy…fingers crossed,*" I said. "*One more thing.*"

"*Yeah?*"

"*No more football players!*"

"*Shit…oh, okay.*"

"*V, I'm serious!*"

"*Fine.*"

I searched high and low for Deylah. No sign of him in the predictable spots, such as his dorm room. Then it occurred to me that he would be out of clothes because of hell week. I ran to the laundry room and, sure enough, there he was, sorting through an enormous pile of clothes. I ogled him from the doorway; he wore his trademark lopsided hat. I could hardly control my breathing or throbbing heart rate.

This is the guy. Don't blow it.

"Hey," I sheepishly said, poking my head through the door frame.

"Did you come by this morning?"

"Yeah," he responded, not looking up from a pair of tube socks. "But it looked like you had company."

Pulling myself together, I strutted into the laundry room and boosted myself up onto an empty dryer.

I need him to look at me if I have any hope of this plan working....

"It didn't mean anything, Deylah," I said in my softest voice. "I didn't think you cared about me. You haven't called in over a week!"

"I couldn't," he explained. "We just crossed this morning, and the first person I came to see was you. Big mistake."

I hopped down and weaseled my body between him and the washing machine. I looked into his eyes. "No. It wasn't a mistake. I'm so sorry. I really didn't think you liked me. I didn't mean to hurt you."

"I'm not hurt, okay? It doesn't matter," he said, shrugging me off and looking away.

"If it doesn't matter, then why did you run out? Why won't you look at me if it doesn't matter? Come on. Just give me another chance. *Please.* I promise it will be different now."

"I don't know," he murmured.

My eyes finally caught his and our gazes locked together. It felt like a dagger cutting into my chest. He was devastated. He looked like he'd lost a loved one. "I need to think about it," he decided.

"Okay, I can live with that…for now," I accepted.

I threw my arms around his neck. His skin was soft and warm. I waited for a moment until I felt him embrace me back.

Touchdown!

FIFTEEN

Hot Wax

DEYLAH AND I SPENT THE REST OF THE SEMESTER TIED AT THE HIP. IN spite of V's pleas, we didn't have sex. I was hellbent on making sure he liked me for more than my body. At the end of May, we said our goodbyes and parted ways for the summer. We endured three long months of writing letters and calling each other by phone before college was back in session and we saw each other again. I missed him terribly the whole time we were apart.

Once the fall semester started, it became clear the two of us still had intense chemistry. His fingertips sent electricity throughout my entire body. I never wanted to leave his side, never mind detach from his lips. I walked around in a perpetual state of arousal when we first started dating—and he did, too. However, I continued to insist that we wait to have sex. I figured we'd made it this far and needed to make sure the moment was perfection.

Deylah gladly accepted my invitation to attend my sorority's Date Night, which was always held at the sorority house. Despite the setting's lack of grandeur, the sisters and I dressed in semiformal gowns and had our hair professionally done. We packed into a car and drove to the top salon in town, where our friends—Candy and Nikki—did the best updos.

I had to look my best because I'd already made an important decision: This was the night Deylah and I were finally going to have sex. That morning, I had shaved my vagina bare to be ready for him. Up until then I had only trimmed and shaved my bikini line but, after hearing a comment on the subject from a frat brother, I figured I better get with the times. Another added benefit, I thought, was that it would help determine whether or not the hair had been getting in the way of the Big O.

This was a big moment for V and me. Luckily, I only nicked myself in two places and they weren't the labia, so the pain was minimal. Mostly V felt cold and exposed; however, my clit had discovered newfound freedom. It was acutely dialed in to every movement, every sensation. It even rubbed against my underwear differently.

"I could get use to this," V said.

As we flew down the highway with "Heads High"—a reggae favorite by Mr. Vegas—blasting on the radio, I shouted, "I'm going to give it up to Deylah tonight!"

Everyone's heads turned toward me.

"What? You haven't screwed him yet?" Kaimbryn asked.

"No," I answered, "I was waiting for a special night."

"Damn, girl. You better get on that," Raelie ordered.

"I know, I know. I'm going to. I just wanted it to be perfect, ya know? Also…I had him get tested for STDs at the health center."

"Really?" all of the girls asked in unison.

"Yeah, I don't really want him to wear a condom—and neither does he. So, he agreed to go."

Raelie stated the obvious: "Damn, bare bones on the first night."

We pulled into the salon parking lot—and not a moment too soon. I was relieved to put a pin in this conversation.

We were greeted by the receptionist, who assigned us to Candy and Nikki. I was up first and hopped in Candy's chair.

"Hey, girl," she said, while planting a kiss on my cheek.

Before I could reply Raelie blurted, "Karin's going to screw Deylah tonight."

"Yay!" Candy applauded, brushing out my hair. "I know just the style for you."

I began to feel at ease as she worked her magic, twisting my hair up and curling the end pieces. I was confident that Candy would make me look hot; my super cute boyfriend would find me irresistible; and the two of us would solidify our relationship with mind-blowing sex.

Thirty minutes later, I sprang out of the chair feeling like a babe. The rest of the girls were done soon after that, and we zoomed back to our dorm rooms to finish getting ready.

I slipped on my black thongs and my beige strapless bra—the hand-me-down from my mom. I immediately regretted being so cheap and not having bought a new one. I prayed the lights would be off by that point, so hopefully he wouldn't notice it.

I pulled out my new black and red lace dress. It was long and touched the floor, covering my short legs. I stepped into my black satin pumps to complete the look and posed in the full-length mirror.

If this doesn't do it, nothing will.

The knock came right on time. I smoothed out my dress and took a deep breath before opening the door.

I could hardly utter a word at the sight of Deylah standing in my doorway holding a single red rose. He had also gone through a transformation to prepare for the evening. He wore a brown leather jacket on top of an oversized white button-down shirt with khaki pants and casual but polished shoes. Best of all: He wasn't wearing his hat, so I was able to get a good look at his hair, which seemingly had been treated with as much affection as mine. The style had a flawless fade. A short buzz at the bottom exposed his slender neck; the hair filled out as it reached the top. The soft brown strands were held together with just the right amount of gel: not too stiff, not too wet.

Wow, he's so hot.

"*Settle down—you still have to get through dinner before you can jump his bones,*" V reminded me.

"Okay, ready to go?"

"Yeah, I'm starving," he blurted.

We decided to walk to the restaurant, even though it was a cold evening and it would take us at least fifteen minutes to get there.

Can't we just skip all of this and go up to his room now?

We entered the fancy Italian restaurant, where the hostess verified our reservation at the front desk and led us to a corner table near a window. We had a beautiful view overlooking the main streetlights. Although the area felt a bit drafty, I removed my coat so he could see my dress.

The waitress dropped a basket full of rolls on the table. I snatched one with the initial intent of nibbling at it. I applied some butter to the roll and bit a corner. Before I knew what was happening, I had devoured the whole thing. I looked down at the crumbs on my plate, unable to process how ravenous I felt.

Whoa, piggy. Slow your roll!

My stomach demanded more and growled, but I fought off the urge in order to leave room for the actual meal. My eyes didn't venture away from the basket full of rolls as Deylah and I placed our orders and then engaged in typical college chitchat: *What's your favorite rap song? How is your Psych class going? When is your next dance performance?*

A few minutes later, the waitress re-emerged and placed a sizable plate of cheese ravioli in front of me. I delicately placed a napkin across my lap.

Deylah, meanwhile, picked up his fork and dug right into his meal.

"*Ahem,*" I snickered. "You should put your napkin on your lap."

I'm a moron—what a turnoff! I probably sound like his mother.

"Oh, right," he obliged.

Dinner was delicious and went off without a hitch. He paid the bill, and we made our way to the sorority house.

On arrival, we climbed up the staircase to the wraparound porch where a handful of sisters and their dates were having a smoke and drinking from either red plastic cups or fancy ones decorated with pledge names. I hadn't earned one of those yet, so I was relegated to drinking from the plain cup.

I grabbed Deylah's hand and guided him to the kitchen, where a group of people stood huddled around the guy who manned a keg. They flashed their empty cups at him. Lucky for me, he happened to be my big sister's boyfriend and had a soft spot for me.

He caught sight of me amidst the crowd and winked, "Little Sis, I got you," before filling my cup. When he was done, I presented him with Deylah's cup: "One more, please."

He graciously filled it. Mission complete!

I played beer pong with my sisters...drank...played the game with Deylah...danced with him in the living room (and on the living room table)...drank...laughed up a storm...and drank some more.

The night couldn't have been going any better, even though it was starting to get fuzzy. It was so loud that I could barely hear Deylah over the music.

"Wanna see the upstairs?"

"If it's quieter, then yes."

"It is quieter and I'm pretty sure it's haunted, so maybe you'll see a ghost."

"Whoa."

We made our way up the staircase and headed down the dim hallway. I was going to show him my pledge class's paddle. When we were midway, he grabbed my hand and spun me around for a kiss. We locked lips for several minutes, during which he pressed me against the wall. I felt the displayed paddles from previous pledges pressing against my back.

Time stopped. When I pulled away to catch a breath, our eyes locked.

"I have total tunnel vision when I'm with you," I babbled.

"I know the feeling," he returned, not caring that I sounded corny and drunk.

"You wanna get out of here?" he asked.

"Definitely."

No doubt he was also thinking about one thing: sex. We said rushed goodbyes and hit the streets. While we were in a hurry to get to the main event, we hadn't yet decided whose room would serve as our setting.

"We can go to my room," I offered. "Raelie won't be back for a while."

"I have another idea," he countered. "My roommate went to Rochester. I thought you could stay overnight in my room."

"Even better!"

We reached his dorm building, where he held the door open for me.

Again, the perfect gentleman....

We stepped inside. No one was in sight.

"Close your eyes," he said as we approached his bedroom door.

"What?"

"You heard me, just do it."

I reluctantly followed his instruction.

"Don't open them until I tell you to."

"I won't," I promised.

I admit that I kept a tiny crack between my lashes open so I wouldn't trip on anything. I heard the flick of a lighter...and waited.

"Okay...you can open them now."

At last, I can look....

Fresh rose petals were arranged on the bed. Candles flickered around the room. He stood in the middle of it all, glowing like an angel from heaven.

Yes, this is the night! He is the right guy.

We were like magnets drawn to each other. My dress flew off in one swift motion.

Damn...he can totally see this crappy bra in this light.

I quickly ditched it, exposing my hard nipples. There was no hiding my arousal at this point. I peered down at his khaki pants; there was no hiding his excitement, either. I undid his belt and pants to free willy. He gently lifted me up, which showed off his biceps.

Ooh, where are we going? I hope I'm not too heavy.

He carried me to his desk and shoved away some papers to make room for my butt. He kissed every inch of my skin from neck to foot.

Is this really happening? I wish I weren't so drunk right now. I want to remember every moment of this.

His lips made their way back up my torso, before removing my underwear.

He was greeted by a bald beaver.

"You *shaved*," he gawked.

He reached behind and grabbed a lit candle and placed it beside us.

Why did he move the candle? To get a better view?

"Lean back," he commanded, guiding himself inside me with ease. Now that my bush had been deforested, he had no trouble hitting his mark. There was no need to worry about my being wet enough; he slid right in.

V floated on a cloud. She had never felt a penis without a condom. Deylah and I had already discussed not using one, since his tests had come back clean. As for risk of pregnancy, we had decided we would take our chances and use the old pullout method.

"*Woo-hoo! Give me some skin!*" V gushed.

He raised the candle and tilted it, allowing a few drops of wax to land between my breasts and near my nipples.

This feels amazing....

He thrust deeper and dripped a bit more wax. Thrust, drip... thrust, drip.

Wow—where did he learn this? I wonder if he does this with all his girlfriends? Ugh, why am I thinking about that right now?

"*Shut up, Karin, and just enjoy!*" V berated me.

The wax was running out, so he placed the candle back on the table. Once again, he picked me up, carrying me toward the bed. He placed me down on the rose petals. They felt cool against my back and smelled amazing. We explored each other's bodies, living in the moment.

About twenty minutes later, he flipped me over for doggystyle, but not before once again reaching for the candle. He applied the hot wax on my back. This time, it burned. I didn't react because I could tell he was enjoying it and I didn't want to spoil the moment.

Maybe the alcohol is wearing off?

Eventually, he ran out of wax and I could focus on pleasure instead of pain. We twisted and tangled into every imaginable position. I was shocked by how long he was lasting—especially considering what had happened the night of our first encounter.

Maybe he drank a lot? Or took care of himself before picking me up?

No matter. It lasted just the right amount of time. He pulled out for his orgasm, and then we crumpled into each other's arms in an exhausted heap.

"That was amazing," he reflected while brushing my hair behind my ear with his fingers.

"Thanks," I teased. "You're not so bad yourself."

Part of me longed to ask about the hot wax and whether he'd done it before, but I couldn't take the chance of killing the mood. Instead, I opted for a kiss. We snuggled with my head on his chest.

My mind replayed our relationship right up until that moment. I was so glad we had waited. The evening had far exceeded my expectations. We were perfect together. V fit him like a glove.

Unfortunately, I still hadn't achieved the mythical Big O. I also had to contend with the morning after…the hangover and the dreaded walk of shame to my dorm in a rumpled gown and my hot-mess hairdo.

On the other hand, I could now check hot wax and raw dog off my bucket list. *Booyah!*

SIXTEEN

Pussy Power!

WHETHER THEY ADMIT IT OR NOT, ALL WOMEN HAVE A SUPERPOWER. Soon after Deylah and I consummated our relationship, I discovered that V was blessed with this special gift. To my delight, I realized she and I didn't need a costume, a golden lasso, or even to get bitten by a radioactive spider in order to tap into this ability.

What is this magical force? *Pussy power!*

Like every superpower, this can be a truly empowering and rewarding asset—if harnessed correctly. (Fans of Spider-Man, aka Peter Parker, will recall his Uncle Ben's charter: "With great power comes great responsibility.")

Most of us are already familiar with the term *pussy-whipped*. If you aren't, here is my definition:

> Being completely under the control of a woman and doing every-
> thing she says; historically, this refers to a man who obeys every
> command from his girlfriend or wife.

A lot of people regard this as a negative term that has sexist con-notations. This is certainly the case when pussy power is misused and a woman takes advantage of it.

I, for one, have never seen anything wrong with a woman acknowledging the greatness of her pussy. I believe that being pussy-whipped is your man's way of conveying to the world how good your lovin' is. So, I say, *the more pussy-whipped a man is, the better!*

For the most part, I have utilized my superpower with appropriate strength and admirable restraint. Unfortunately, there were also those occasions in which I failed to heed the "With great power comes great responsibility" refrain.

There was one set of circumstances, in particular....

ⓖⓢⓐ

Like many college sweethearts, Deylah—or Damien, as I now referred to him by his birth name—and I went through our fair share of on-again, off-again spurts. Junior year started off great until I had an itch to travel and see the world. I had heard about our university's semester abroad program and became intrigued. Unsure of whether I would be accepted anywhere, I applied to schools in three places: Kingston, Jamaica; Middlesex, England; and Adelaide, Australia.

The letters arrived three weeks later. To my astonishment, all three had green lighted me. I couldn't wait to share the news with Damien. I knew he had an African Dance class at Hartwell Hall until 4:30, so I planned to meet him at the exit of that building. (And yes, he took African Dance; someone told him it was a great way to meet girls. Perhaps he feared we might not last....)

I was about fifty feet away from the Hartwell entrance when I saw him step out the door. As always, he was wearing his blue Detroit cap backwards. He had on a sweatshirt and a pair of track pants.

I froze at the sight of him: The reality of studying abroad and being without him for a full semester suddenly hit me full blast. My heart ached, which caused me to sprint full throttle toward him. "I got in! I got into all three schools!" I shouted.

He stretched out his long arms and bent down to scoop me up. His hands cupped my butt as he twirled me in a circle with our faces pressed together. I already missed him....

"I knew you would—congratulations!"

He kissed me on the lips and gently lowered me. "So...where are you going to go?"

"I don't know," I shrugged, still breathless from running and being spun. "I need to talk to my parents. I haven't even told them yet...I wanted you to be the first to know."

Damien seemed genuinely happy for me. The next few weeks, neither of us was prepared to bring up the issue of our looming physical separation. We carried on as if everything was perfectly normal.

During that time, I decided to accept the program at University of Adelaide in Australia. I figured that it was so far away I might never get another opportunity to visit that country on my own. Besides, I reasoned, they had a superb Dance program.

As my departure drew nearer, I began to think a lot about my relationship with Damien. We were young and in love, but we had a lot of living to do. I didn't want to tie him down while I was gone, or worse, for either of us to get lonely and cheat. I decided that it was best for us to go our separate ways. If we wanted to get back together when I returned for senior year, then all the better. At that point, we'd know whether we were truly meant to be.

Just one problem: How was I going to break the news to him? Little by little, I tried to distance myself from him. I didn't return calls. We didn't go to classes together. I told him I was busy with sorority duties when I wasn't. I even withheld sex.

This was awful. I was gently peeling off the bandage and prolonging the pain, instead of ripping it off with one swipe.

I knew I couldn't procrastinate any further; I had to deliver the blow. I donned my best outfit: a black ASA long-sleeved shirt, Mudd jeans, and a white Ruff Ryders bandana, which I fashioned into a headband by tying a knot at the back of my neck. I steeled myself in the mirror to summon up courage.

Before I knew it, I was sitting on a black futon in his living room with the lights dimmed. He was up close beside me. I pressed my lips together, unsure of where to begin.

"You know I love you, right?" I mustered.

"If you love me so much, why have you been ignoring me?"

"You know I'm leaving, Damien. I'm going to be in another country. It's not fair to either of us."

His lips quivered but he refused to blink. He stared me down with his big brown eyes. "I don't want to break up," he declared.

Shit. This bandage is stuck tight.

"We don't have a choice," I blurted. "I'll be far away for a really long time."

He folded his arms, obstinate. "Well, I'm not going anywhere. I'm here now, and I'm going to be right here when you get back."

He lifted my chin with his finger and moved in for a kiss.

This is not a good idea. But it tastes and feels so wonderful...I don't want this to end.

His hand worked its way through my hair as he held my head close to him for as long as I'd allow.

If I kiss him any longer, I'll end up staying. We'll have sex one last time, which will only make things even harder.

I broke away from his embrace. We fell silent, lost in an abyss of sadness. And, just like that, our relationship came to an end.

⊚⊚⊚

The following weekend, my friend Martina came to visit me in Brockport. We went out for a big night on the town. Newly single, we danced the night away at a local bar, guzzled beers, and flirted with guys. It didn't take long before we were smashed. In my sorry state, I came up with an idea.

"We should check in on Damien," I suggested.

"Sure!" Martina concurred.

Damien had recently broken his leg while riding his bike and required surgery. I felt bad for him, especially since I hadn't seen him since the accident. I merrily led the way through a back alley to Damien's apartment. As we approached his door, I had a brief moment of clarity. "This is a bad idea. Don't let me have sex with him, okay?"

"Yeah, yeah. I got your back. Should we have a code word?"

"Like what? *Pizza* or something?"

"I was thinking more along the lines of...*dry panties* or *chastity belt*."

"How on earth am I going to casually work that into a sentence?"

"Fine. *Pizza*, then."

"Good," I finalized. "If I say, 'I could go for some pizza,' that's your cue to force me out of there."

"Got it," she registered, leaning her shoulder on the door to prop herself up.

The door opened and Martina went down like a pile of bricks. At least she had the decency to land with her legs crossed. I burst out laughing as Austin, Damien's roommate, tried to figure out what had just happened.

"Hi, Austin...this is Martina, my friend from high school. She drank...*a lot*."

"No kidding," Austin remarked.

I stepped over Martina to enter the apartment. "Is Damien here? How's he doin'?"

"He's in his room," Austin answered, struggling to lift Martina up. "Watch out, though, he's in a shitty mood. You want a beer before you go back?"

"Nah—not unless you want me laid out on your floor, too."

Austin guided Martina over to the futon, where she faded in and out of consciousness.

"I'll be right back," I said to her. "I'm just going to check on Damien."

"Okay!" Martina shouted, winking at me. "Just let me know if you're hungry and want to get some *pizza!*"

I tried to compose myself as I made my way to Damien's door. I knocked while simultaneously opening it. He was lying on his bed watching TV; as expected, his leg was in a cast and raised on a couple of pillows.

And then...I phased out, most likely from the last shot at the bar. This still occurred from time to time, even after I got rid of the medicine. Once again, V turned on autopilot while my brain was on hiatus.

When I snapped out of it, I found myself riding up and down on Damien.

"Whoo-hoo!" V cheered. *"Back in the saddle again!"*

Holy shit, holy shit—what am I doing? Pizza! Pizza! Pizza!

Perplexed, I focused on Damien's face. I'd never seen him this blissfully happy.

"I can't do this to him, V! I'm such an asshole."

"It's fine. This dude is pussy-whipped. He seems pretty glad we stopped by!"

I knew it was past time for me to take charge.

"Um...I totally forgot about Martina," I bleated, patting his chest. "Gotta go!"

I don't know why, but I sang Britney Spears as I hopped off him: *"Oops!...I did it again."* I slid on my underwear on, fixed my skirt, and grabbed my purse off his dresser.

Poor guy. He doesn't know what hit him.

I hightailed it out of the room—leaving Damien with nothing but blue balls to show for my visit—and grabbed Martina on the futon. "Come on, we need *pizza!*"

"Were you just having sex with him?" Austin asked as we tripped our way out.

"Bye, Austin!" I shouted. "And...yes, I was!"

Phew. Made it out alive...barely.

Fortunately, it wasn't long before the semester ended, and I was off to Australia. V and I were by now both well aware of the fact that we couldn't be anywhere near Damien. Beyond a shadow of doubt, I was just as whipped by his penis as he was by my pussy.

SEVENTEEN

Down Under

My semester abroad at Adelaide University in Australia began with disappointment. The school lost its Dance program to a competing college and couldn't offer any related classes to me. They gave me an opportunity to cancel, but I hadn't signed up for any classes at SUNY Brockport, so I didn't have much choice. I decided to turn my Business minor into a major and change courses accordingly.

Aussie boys, here I come!

Upon landing in Adelaide Airport, my fellow exchange students and I were driven to Lincoln College, the location of my dorm room. If you're confused, join the club. In Australia at that time, students attended a university (in my case, Adelaide) but lived at a college (such as Lincoln). Sports activities and most clubs were at the college, not the university.

Obviously, I had a lot of adjustments to make in Australia—but not all of them were bad. For starters, I didn't have a roommate, which gave me lots of privacy.

When it comes to drinking, Australians surpass their reputations. I thought I had seen some pretty impressive drinkers on American campuses, but Aussies take this to a whole new level. My first day on campus, a Coopers truck pulled up. The roll-up door swung open to reveal several kegs. Everyone was handed a beer mug that was filled to the brim. And it was *free!*

The partying spree had begun.

At one of many such parties, a couple of girlfriends and I were minding our business and enjoying our beers when a few local gentlemen struck up a conversation with us. I was flirtatious by nature but didn't see much of interest at this point and broke away from the group.

My girlfriends were baffled. "Karin, that guy was *hot!* Why did you just walk away?" Katie assailed me.

What have I done?

"*You just blew my chance at a true blue Aussie, that's what you've done,*" V berated me.

"I'll take him if you don't want him," Katie jumped in.

If my friends and V think he's hot, then maybe he is?

That settled it. I decided right then and there that he was going to be my next conquest. The hunt was on for my friends to help me find this mystery man. We darted through what seemed like hundreds of students until Katie nudged at my back with her knuckles. "Found him—twelve o'clock," she gestured.

I turned my head to refresh my memory of this so-called hottie.

Check, check, check, and check: Tall, slender, golden brown hair, and chiseled jaw. Just my type. How could I have misjudged him?

I waited for him to flash a smile while conversing with his friend. I'd already discovered the vital importance of this. My first week in the country, I had approached a beautiful Aussie boy who also checked all of the boxes. When he opened his mouth to laugh, his exposed teeth were more jagged than the Great Barrier Reef. Instant turnoff.

His expression widened, revealing a fine set of pearly whites. I set my sights on my prey, who towered over me.

"Oh, hey there," I intervened. "We meet again."

"I wondered where you ran off to," he crooned.

"*Ooh…that accent,*" V melted.

"Do you always play this hard to get?"

"Not always," I teased, slipping my arm around his waist. "I'm here now. What's your name?"

"Billy. What's yours?"

"Karin—with an *i*, not an *e*."

"I like it—sounds exotic."

Seriously? I've never thought of my name that way before.

I drank, chatted, and flirted with Billy and his mates, and we all became fast friends.

"Want to go to the club?" one of the guys suggested.

I huddled with my collegemates to come to a consensus. It didn't take much time for us to agree that it would be great fun to hang out with local Australians on their own turf. We drove off to the club, where we danced and continued the party. Twenty minutes after arriving, the DJ announced a contest: The girl who could lick the most jelly off a random guy's stomach would win.

I don't know whether it was V or me who set our ball in motion, but whatever the case, I tossed it out there. "Hold my beer, Billy," I commanded.

"Where are you going?" he asked with concern.

"I'm gonna win this contest," I boasted.

I shot him a deviant wink as my leg slipped over the silver bars that separated the dance floor from the bar area. I weaved through the crowd and hoisted myself up on stage.

Billy and the other guys were stunned, to say the least.

If my jelly-licking skills don't seal the deal with Billy, nothing will.

The DJ announced the details of the contest. Jelly was smeared on the stomachs of the contestants. The buzzer sounded. I set to work, frantically licking jelly off this stranger's stomach.

I was in mid-lick when a hand grabbed mine and threw it in the air.

"The winner!" the DJ proclaimed. I was met with deafening cheers, applause, and whistles.

Imagine…me…jelly-licking queen! What an accomplishment!

My tongue officially become the most sought-after body part in the club. I stared out into the sea of blackness and tried to spot Billy, but the stage lights blinded me. I was awarded several drink tickets and pranced off the stage like Annie Oakley having claimed victory at a shooting match.

"Holy crap—that was *amazing!*" shouted Peter, one of Billy's friends. "You sure picked a feisty one, Billy!"

Billy laughed, his cheeks having turned bright red. I couldn't tell if he was turned on or embarrassed by me. "The next round is on me!" I exclaimed, waving my free drink tickets.

A couple of hours later, the bartender signaled last call. Now it was time to find out if my hard work had paid off.

"All I can say is, I hope Billy hops into my pouch!" V prodded.

As we went to his flat to allow the evening to play out, a fleeting thought of Damien popped into my head. I successfully submerged it by thinking about how fun new romances can be. There is a certain suspense involved. Couples take their time, feeling out what the other person likes and will respond to.

Billy and I made out on his bed for what seemed like hours—kissing, fondling, and rolling around. Music from his stereo system became our soundtrack, dictating every move. We removed our shirts and pressed up against each other. My pants went down, followed by his.

Hmn, something different here than usual….

He was definitely erect, but something seemed a bit off. The tip of his member didn't jab into my leg the way other penises had. I paid little attention as my head moved south.

I inched my hands down his legs and slid off his boxers. I looked closer to inspect the goods and align it with my mouth. It was dark but my eyesight gradually adjusted to the cracks of moonlight shining through his blinds. I had to rub my eyes to believe what I was seeing.

Halt! Can it be? Is this…an uncircumcised penis? Oh, shit. What do I do?

This was a foreign land with so much uncharted territory.

Where is the tip? Maybe I should use my hands first.

I hesitantly gripped the shaft with my hand.

Feels like a normal penis.

I used my hand to slide back the extra fold of skin that hid the tip.

I hope this doesn't hurt him.

Like a turtle coming out his shell, the tip popped out to greet me.

No way. Foreskin...forget it!

I honestly didn't know what to make of this.

Is this thing clean? Aren't uncircumcised penises prone to infections? Are all Aussie guys like this down there?

"What are you waiting for?" V interrogated.

"I don't know if I can do this, V. I don't want to hurt his feelings, but this is weird."

"It's college, you're supposed to do weird stuff. That's why they call it the 'old college try.' Suck it up, buttercup."

Here goes nothing....

My tongue steered clear of the tip, just to be on the safe side. Turns out—circumcised or not, all men come too quickly. The evening was over.

Well, at least one of us has been satisfied!

However, I couldn't help but feel as if I'd gained something from the experience, too. I had a good story to tell about the jelly licking and my having unveiled Billy's uncircumcised penis. It was as if I had discovered a rare gem.

One might think this unusual sexual encounter would be relegated to a one-night stand. Not so! Billy was a romantic and exuded a maturity that I hadn't experienced with other guys my age. He called the next day and asked me out on a coffee date that upcoming Friday.

A coffee date? Never been on one of those. Sounds sophisticated!

I suppose I was also curious to see what else the hooded warrior had in store for me.

We met at a place called the Elephant Walk Cafe, where we were seated at a cute booth for two with curtains draped all around it. I felt as if I was in a Middle Eastern palace: surrounded by vibrant colors and fabrics with exotic music piped into our booth. Something about this adult experience was turning me on, and we hadn't even ordered anything yet.

The conversation turned intellectual. Billy shared his aspirations for a career in business, as well as his views on current events. I wondered how I was faring as we sipped our drinks. I began to become more comfortable when he asked me several personal questions, granting me the spotlight. A good listener always scores some points.

This time—loaded up with caffeine rather than alcohol—we headed to his place. After a sufficient amount of chitchat, he flicked the light switch. It became like the clichéd movie sex scene in which two people can't keep their hands off each other and clothes fly into the air. I hoped the evening wouldn't end as abruptly as last time.

He seemed intent on making sure I didn't leave without a parting gift. He rolled me over onto my back and climbed on top. Our eyes met. He slinked down under the covers. I bit my lip and let my eyes drift up to the ceiling. V began to purr. And then….

"Bloody ripper!"[1] V howled in delight.

That evening, Billy earned his nickname: the Tongue Master. At the time, V discovered that few men truly know what they are doing down there. My Aussie boy was one of the greats! He had a tongue of steel that never tired. He could have gone on forever—or at least the remaining two months of my stay.

For all of the pleasure V and I received from the Tongue Master, the Big O continued to elude us. But he made my study abroad even more memorable and proved conclusively that men from Down Under really know how to *go down*.

---

[1] Translation: Aussie for "Really awesome!"

EIGHTEEN

Fire Crotch

On my return to the States, I regrouped with my boy from Queens. You might be wondering if he was mad about my time with Billy in Australia. To a degree, yes, but it's not like he was a saint while I was away, either. (I doubt he did much in the way of jelly licking, however.)

Valentine's Day. I wanted this to be special for Damien, so I ventured into Frederick's of Hollywood for the first time. The lingerie was a lot racier than at Victoria's Secret, which I had frequented in the past. Once I arrived there and tried things on, I chickened out and went for the tamest thing in the store: a red lace teddy and black thigh high stockings to match. While I was checking out, the woman at the counter recommended I try some chocolate body butter. I didn't have a clue what do with it, but it sounded intriguing and, at eight dollars, was just the right price, so I had the cashier ring it up.

That evening, I donned my new outfit for Damien and we went at it. The chocolate butter, which he smeared all over my body—including V—was icing on the cake. Without getting into too many details, let's just say he became ravenous.

The following morning, I woke up late and went to pee in my filthy sorority house bathroom. As I sat there with my pajama pants around my knees and my flip-flops sticking to the beer-soaked floor, an unusual sensation spread throughout V unlike anything we'd ever felt.

"*I've got a bad feelin' about this,*" she fretted.

"*I'm sure it's nothing, it'll pass,*" I comforted her.

As the seconds passed, I began to feel less confident in my assurances. It wasn't pain, exactly, but it wasn't pleasure, either. It troubled me that I couldn't tell the difference. At best, it could only be described as feeling like something burned. Yet, I felt like I might climax at the same time (even though I hadn't experienced the Big O).

I checked my watch: 12:28 PM. Thirty-two minutes until my Ballet class. I didn't have nearly enough time for a visit to the infirmary and get my issue checked out.

Fine. I'll deal with it later. How bad can it be?

"*That's easy for you to say!*" V blurted.

I had just enough time to freshen myself up in my bedroom. I slipped on my leotard and tights. I moved to the mirror to wrap my hair in a bun when I was overcome by another uncontrollable urge to pee.

Huh. I just went!

"*You better get our butt back over there,*" V warned.

I raced to the bathroom, plunked myself down, and...out came a spittle.

"*Sorry about that,*" V apologized. "*I don't know what's going on around here. Maybe your lover-boy gave us a surprise gift—one that keeps giving.*"

Oh no, an STD? That bastard! I swear, I'll kill him. He probably got it from that girl he hooked up with while I was in Australia—whore! What do I do now?

I remained determined to get to my class on time. I finished up in the bathroom and returned to my room, where I grabbed my purse and a bag of chips to eat on the way. Oddly, even though I lived in a house full of women, I was too embarrassed to tell anyone about what I was experiencing.

I made it to Ballet in the nick of time. I threw my bag in a cubby and ran to find an open spot at the barre. I took a deep breath, hoping I could get through class without the problem becoming exacerbated. We began with a routine of pliés and grand pliés.

Perfect: five minutes down, fifty-five to go.

By the time we started on grand battements—think high kicks—things took a turn for the worse. The urge to pee came back with a vengeance. This didn't make any sense; I hadn't had a thing to drink since leaving the sorority house.

I don't have to pee, I don't have to pee, I don't have to pee.

I swung my right leg straight up in front of me and quickly pulled it back in. In doing so, I thought I felt a squirt of pee release.

One more movement and there is going to be a puddle on this dance floor.

It would be an understatement to say I was in a panic. This felt like life and death. I decided to do "smaller" grand battements with my legs squeezed together as much as possible.

It's working—no one noticed!

Unfortunately, I wasn't quite as successful cheating the movement when my leg went to the back—especially since this had become my specialty.

"Higher, Karin! You're slacking off!" the teacher scolded me.

Busted! I had no option except to kick higher on the next attempt. Despite an effort to tilt my back forward to prevent my legs from spreading too wide, I couldn't tighten my muscles enough to keep V closed.

Meanwhile, my teacher—who looked like Fabio from the "I Can't Believe It's Not Butter!" commercials—floated across the floor toward me, his long hair wafting behind him. Suddenly, he was right beside me, holding his hand in the air at the spot he expected me to kick. I had no choice except to kick his hand and pray that a geyser didn't shoot out of V onto him.

I think…something came out. Does he know? My leotard is maroon; it'll look darker if it's wet.

"Much better," he praised without flinching. "Don't let me see you lean forward again, either." I forced a smile, hoping he wouldn't bother me again.

I sprang to the bathroom during the next water break. The dire need to go had again become overwhelming. I was relieved to discover that I hadn't peed myself but dismayed when only a few drops tinkled out. Then….

V: *Help, I'm burning up!*
V and me: *Emergency, 911—call the fire department!*

By the time I returned to the studio, the other dancers were lined up on the far side of the room to move across the floor. I had to brave the entire area with everyone staring at me. I felt like I was back in high school cheerleading practice battling an ovarian cyst. Except…this couldn't possibly have been a cyst. It was unlikely that this dance teacher was going to be as understanding as my cheerleading coach.

"Something important happen out in the hall, Karin? Would you care to share why you're late?"

"No, sir, sorry about that."

"Ladies, this is only a one-hour class. I need you to be focused for the duration. Are we clear?"

The entire room responded, "Yes, sir."

I wanted to hide under a rock. Since one wasn't available, I slinked behind Liz, one of my sorority sisters.

"What's up with you today?" she asked. "Rough night or something?"

Should I tell her? Maybe she has some advice for me?

"I have to pee all the time. When I go, hardly anything comes out."

"That's weird."

"Yeah, I know. Now it's *burning*. I can't explain it."

"Shit, maybe you got an STD?"

"That's what I thought. I swear, I'll kill Damien if I do," I snarled.

"Ladies!" the teacher barked.

Nabbed again.

"Is there something you'd like to share with the whole class?"

Cut me some slack, man! I'm in agony here. Any other day, I could tolerate you riding my ass in front of the whole class—but not today, buddy.

"Yeah, I've got something to share all right," I broke down. "An STD, I think…maybe. I don't know…but I gotta pee again."

What have I just admitted in front of the entire class and my male teacher?

The poor guy was speechless. What could he possibly have said?

I can't take any more. I need the ladies' room—bad.

Accompanied by the sound of girls snickering, I marched across the floor, out of the room, and back to the ladies' room.

Afterward, I waited in the hall for the remaining hour of the class. I was way too embarrassed to return to the room and look anyone in the face.

Me and my big mouth! What if I do have an STD and everyone on campus finds out about it? Worse yet, what if it isn't a venereal disease and people think I have one anyway?

When the class ended and everyone streamed into the hallway, I called out to my sorority sister: "Liz!"

She didn't mince words as she approached me: "What the fuck was that?"

"I don't know. I just freaked out. I'm really stressed right now," I admitted. "But I need a favor. Can you get my bag from the cubby? I can't go back in there."

"Sure, one sec."

When she returned with my bag, I thanked her and said, "I'm going to the infirmary to get this checked out. I'll see you back at the house. Oh, and let's keep this little outburst between us. Okay?"

"Good luck! I hope you don't have chlamydia or anything."

"Gee, thanks—me too."

As it happens, I did not have an STD at all. Damien was off the hook, and I was glad that I hadn't been given a chance to rip him a new one.

The diagnosis? A UTI—urinary tract infection.

The likely cause? The combination of chocolate body butter and not having peed after intercourse. As I discovered, the latter is essential when it comes to UTI prevention. Why hadn't my mom ever taught me such things?

V and me: *At least it's not an STD!*

The infirmary medical team advised me to drink lots of water and cranberry juice. I was given a prescription for an antibiotic and told not to have sex for three days.

V and me: *Three days!*

To my surprise, Damien was totally cool about holding off for a few days. He even used some of his dining points to buy me Ocean Spray cranberry juice from the campus dining hall.

What a guy. I'll never doubt him again...as long as we keep the fire out of my hole!

NINETEEN

Lights, Camera, Action!

HAVE YOU EVER DREAMED ABOUT BEING ON THE BIG SCREEN OR starring in your own television show? When I was in college, I was obsessed with the then-popular MTV show *Diary*. I wanted nothing more than to be a worldwide celebrity and have my own episode. While I did manage to get my moment in front of the camera, it wasn't exactly what I'd expected.

One evening, after a night of drinking at a local bar without Damien (he hadn't yet managed to obtain a fake ID), I went to his apartment to spend the night. I loved it there because he had a king-sized bed and a skylight in the ceiling. Nothing makes a woman feel more alive than looking up at the stars while being enveloped by her dream boy.

I also hated his apartment for several reasons. First, there was the matter of his scattered mess, which included a tripod for one of his Communications classes. (Like so many other college students struggling to pick a major, he'd chosen this field as his fallback.) Then there were his loud roommates and friends, who would some-times accidentally walk in on us while we were...busy.

Accident. Yeah. Right.

In any case, the pros outweighed the cons, and I made myself feel at home. I always had my grungy, shredded tee-shirt waiting there for me to wear to bed and a spare toothbrush.

When I arrived at Damien's apartment, he sat in the center of his bed smoking a Newport with a black light on. He smiled, flashing a set of glowing white teeth but otherwise not moving a muscle. I bummed a cigarette from him before flinging off my platform heels and crawling beside him on the bed.

I filled him in on my antics at the bar as we puffed on our cigarettes. We kissed in between stories. "Do you want your tee-shirt?" he asked, releasing me.

"Yeah, I can't wait to ditch this bra," I replied.

As he fetched my shirt, I took notice of the video camera on his desk. "Someday I want to be on *Diary*," I ruminated, imagining myself as a celebrity on the show.

A forerunner of reality TV, *Diary* featured stars such as Britney Spears, Aaliyah, and Jennifer Love Hewitt, who were willing to reveal their private lives on camera for a few days as they went about their regular business. The program started out by saying, "You think you know, but you have no idea. This is the *Diary* of [insert celebrity name]."

Damien flung my shirt at me and snickered, "I'd watch that."

I grabbed the camera and set it up on the edge of his dresser. I pulled off my blouse and bra but did not replace them with the tee-shirt. Instead, I pressed the record button and posed into the camera while seated at the edge of the bed.

"You think you know, but you have no idea. This is the diary of Karin Freeland," I teased.

The next thing I knew, Damien was showering me with kisses. We were well aware the camera was still rolling but pretended to be oblivious. At the time, it didn't register that we were doing something pornographic.

Our normal activities ran their course—except that, at least from my perspective, it felt a lot more titillating than usual.

V seemed to relish the spotlight: *"I'm ready for my close-up, Mr. DeMille!"*

Our home video drew to its natural conclusion, and Damien rose to clean himself up. Before he returned to me, he turned the camera off. "Guess we don't need that on anymore," he said.

After a slight pause he timidly proposed an idea: "So…wanna watch it?"

"Yeah," I affirmed, trying to be cool despite my nervousness. "What's the point of making a video if you aren't going to watch it?"

"I hope we look hot," V remarked. *"I don't wanna see any roast beef."*

V's concerns compounded my own self-consciousness.

What if I look stupid?

I put my tee-shirt on while Damien hooked the camera up to the TV. Cigarettes in hand, we snuggled up to watch our intimate lovemaking.

We had inadvertently recorded the scene in night mode, which meant it was all set in black and white. I counted my blessings for this as the action commenced.

It started out sweet and slow. We looked remarkably tender. I enjoyed watching how he held me and sweetly touched my back and neck. At first, it was rated R without that much to see, as I was on top of him and the covers blocked key body parts.

"We have no showmanship," I complained to V.

"Well, you're the one hogging up the camera!" she countered. *"But… from what's there, we look pretty damn good!"*

She was right. Objectively speaking, we *did* look good in spite of the fact that we seemed to be hiding from the camera and the film probably wouldn't have made it to the amateur aisle of a third-rate porn shop.

All of a sudden, *boom!* Quick cut—and it was all there, front and center: Every in and out thrust.

"Whoa!" V exclaimed. *"Get the popcorn! Look at my wide smile…. Hey, I'm getting' excited again. Maybe we need to do some retakes!"*

The more Damien and I looked, however, the more we cringed. The sight of his hairy butt and my haphazardly shaved beaver in motion looked absurd. Damien and I turned to each other, laughing hysterically.

"*Hey! You laughin' at me?!*" V complained.

"Maybe we should fast-forward this part?" I suggested.

"That's a good idea."

"*No! Don't!*" V protested. "*I want to see how this flick turns out—I'm the protagonist!*"

Damien pressed the fast-forward button. We watched our movements speed up as a blur, which was even funnier than before.

"You know we have to erase this!" I exclaimed.

"We'll see," he leered.

I hit him, letting him know he didn't have an option. The last thing I needed was his roommates—or worse, his classmates—stumbling across the video.

"Wait a minute," Damien considered, allowing the video to play. "I want to see this part."

Of course he did. We had switched to doggystyle, which no male can seem to resist ogling.

As it turned out, I couldn't take my eyes off the screen, either. Damien's arm muscles seemed to have more definition on camera than in real life. I don't know whether it was the camera angle or lighting but seeing him like this gave me a whole new appreciation for his body. My heart fluttered.

We watched the remainder up to the denouement and climax.

"*Now I need a cigarette,*" V swooned.

"That was fun!" Damien declared. "I think we should save it."

"Save it? Are you nuts?"

"Do you think I want anyone to see it, either? It's just for us. You have my word."

"Okay," I reluctantly conceded. "As long as you promise to never show it to anyone."

"Don't worry. I'll take the tape out and hide it, so no one ever sees it."

To this day, I still have the tape—and no one else has seen it (or ever will). At least not until I die and my children rummage through my things and discover it. Believing it is a sweet home video, they will pop it in the machine and press play. Boy, will they be in for a shock from beyond the grave!

TWENTY

A Force of Nature

I DON'T KNOW ABOUT YOUR PARENTS, BUT MINE HAD STRICT RULES about guys not sleeping in the same bed—or even room—with me until marriage. Even though Damien and I had spent countless nights together in the college dorm, my sorority house, and elsewhere, he was always relegated to the couch in my parents' house. My dad would always assert, "My house, my rules. When you have your own house, you can do what you like."

During a semester break, Damien stayed at my house for one night on his way back to Queens. Since my house was halfway between Brockport and Queens, it was a convenient place for him to stop off while also providing some extra time for us to be together.

We spent the night out barhopping with my friends before going back to my house and passing out on the couch, which was technically against the rules. We both knew this was dangerous, but the alcohol clouded our judgement.

The next morning, having awoken with a hefty hangover, we showered (separately of course) and dressed. My mom made us a late breakfast, even though she was well aware of our couch stunt and not too pleased. She was glad to have me home and didn't want to start a fight on my first day back.

Moments after breakfast, the house was vacant except for us.

Alone at last! All bets are off.

"Wanna go upstairs?" I suggested.

"Yeah, sure," he answered. "I'll grab a condom from my bag."

"Hurry up!" I pressed.

I ran upstairs ahead of him to clear off my bed and make room for us. I was barely finished with my task when Damien charged at me and threw me on the bed.

Damien paused, breathing heavily: "We have to be *quick*. I don't want your dad coming home early to check on us."

"Don't worry," I assured him. "No one is coming home."

He *was* worried, though, which meant settling for a quickie. No foreplay on the menu for either of us. We tussled off our fresh clothes until he balked when I began to remove my shirt.

"Leave it on," he whispered.

He fumbled with the condom for a few moments and then announced, "There—got it. Here I come!"

Our hasty exchange was all about him getting off, and I was okay with it on this occasion. If I happened to enjoy myself, then lucky me. When he was close to finishing, I unleashed a deep moan and sucked on his ear lobe to send him over the edge.

He collapsed on my body. I struggled to breathe as his dead weight sank into me.

"That was great," he puffed, raising his chest.

Now that my lungs were able to take in fresh oxygen, I smiled and gave him a kiss.

"We don't even have to worry about cleanup," he said.

"I know. You can just throw the condom out in a plastic bag."

"*Oh no!*" I gasped as he withdrew from me.

"What?"

He stared down at himself and the realization sank in. "*Oh, shit.*"

"*Move, move!*" I exclaimed, scissoring my right leg up over his head in a ninja move. I cupped my hand over my vulva as I flung the door open and dashed to the bathroom. I planted my tush on the toilet and peed.

Dear God—why did his condom have to break?!

"Karin—you okay?" he asked through the door. "I'm so sorry! I don't know what happened." After a brief pause, he called to me again: "What are you going to do?"

"I don't know. I need to think. Give me a minute."

I grabbed sheets of toilet paper to wipe myself clean. As soon as I thought I was good to go, another drip came out. I'd never had anyone come inside me before; this was uncharted waters.

How long is this going to last? It's like Niagara Falls down there.

I finally pulled myself together and took a pantyliner from my mom's stash, figuring that it might help soak up whatever was still leaking. When I stepped out of the bathroom, Damien presented me with my underwear and pants.

"Thanks," I said, before slapping him in the chest.

"What was that for?"

"*Because*," I spat. "What are we going to do if I get pregnant? I *can't* get pregnant. No one wants to watch a pregnant dancer!"

"Can't you take one of those pills? You know, the one that makes you not get pregnant."

"I guess…but how do I get one?"

"How should I know?"

Then it hit me: *the hospital.* It was conveniently located right by Applebee's. I could swing by right before work. I picked up shifts as a hostess at Applebee's whenever I was home from college.

"I have a plan—but we have to move quickly."

He shoved his things in his overnight bag, left the house, and dove into his Honda CRX. He sadly waved goodbye to me from the window before driving off. This was certainly not how we had anticipated our final hour together.

I flung on my Applebee's outfit, grabbed my purse, raced into my car, and sped off to the hospital.

I didn't know which part of the hospital to enter but figured I should start off with the emergency room.

"Can I help you, dear?" the receptionist asked.

"Well...um...I...have a little emergency," I began, lowering my voice. "My boyfriend's condom broke and I need one of those pills—the Plan B, I think it's called."

"I see," she registered. "Here is the form. Have a seat and fill this out. We'll be with you in a bit."

"Okay, but...how long is 'a bit'?" I asked, pointing to the logo on my tee-shirt, "I have to be at my hostess job—Applebee's at three."

"We'll do our best. Just bring me the form when it's complete."

I took the first available seat and started filling out the form. Right away I encountered some trouble; there were spaces for parent's name, phone number, policy holder....

Oh no. Are they going to call my parents? They can't do that—can they? I must have some patient confidentiality here.

I returned to the receptionist. "Hi again," I began. "The form is asking me for my parents' information...but I don't want them to know I'm here. Do I have to fill this out?"

"Well, yes," she answered. "You have to pay for the visit, and we'll need your insurance information. If it's under your parents' name, we require their information in order to file the claim."

"Uh-uh," my head shook. "They can't find out about this....."

Tears formed in my eyes. I became choked up, making it difficult to continue to speak. "Look...I just need the pill. It was...an accident. We were being safe.... We...used a condom. I don't know how it broke. *Please*...I need your help."

"Let me get a nurse," she conceded. "Take a seat. There are some tissues on the table."

"Thank you," I sniffled, turning to grab a few tissues.

A few moments later, a nurse appeared and led me into a private room. "Tell me what happened," she said while jotting notes on a clipboard.

"Well, my boyfriend and I were having sex," I explained. "We've been together for almost four years, and we were using a condom and everything. But it broke and his…you know, got all inside me! I tried to pee it out, but I'm afraid some may already have made it to the egg. I really need the Plan B pill. Can you just give it to me?"

"Okay," she nodded. "This was consensual sex?"

"Yes, consensual…like I said, the condom broke. You don't understand! I can't get pregnant—I'm a dance major."

"Well, regardless of major, you can get pregnant if you're sexually active…."

No shit, Sherlock.

"…and I can't just give you the Plan B pill."

"Why not?" I demanded.

The tears poured down. I couldn't understand why she didn't seem to want to help me.

"We're a *Catholic* hospital," she informed me. "We aren't allowed to give out the pill."

Just my luck—I've chosen the only religious hospital in the area.

"I'm not a slut. It was an accident!" I shouted.

"No one accused you of being a slut," she argued. "What we *can* do is have you go through a rape exam, which takes about two hours. We can give you the pill after that."

"But I wasn't raped," I insisted. "I had sex with my boyfriend, whom I love very much. I'll probably marry him someday."

"I understand, but this is the only way we can get around it," she said. "I have to warn you: The exam is a bit…invasive."

"No," I declined. "I don't want a rape exam. I don't want that to appear on any documents. I wasn't raped."

"Well, that's all I can do."

At this point, my brain lost focus and I started rambling. "I have to be at work at 3:00—I don't even have time to do the rape kit thing. What am I supposed to tell my boss, anyway? 'Sorry I'm late. I just fucked my boyfriend and his steroid sperm shot through the condom and fertilized my egg. Then I had to go to the hospital and get a rape exam, even though it was consensual, to get the Plan B.'"

She remained calm as she stated, "I understand your frustration, dear—but these are the consequences of having sex before marriage."

Yeah, I got that. Bitch.

"Thanks for making me feel like a whore," I fired back, snatching the paperwork out of her hand and marching out of the hospital. Once safely in my car, I sat and cried.

Why, God? I didn't mean for this to happen. I don't want to be pregnant. Please, please, please, don't let me be pregnant. We were trying to be safe. Clearly, it's the condom's faulty design to blame!

Regaining my composure, I reached into the glove box for my makeup bag. I looked like a vampire in a thunderstorm. I had some serious touching up to do. I flipped down the sunshade mirror to get a better image of myself when a photograph of Damien and me dropped into my lap.

I stared at it for several minutes, knowing damn well there was no one else I would want to father my child—if I were to be pregnant, that is. The corners of my mouth perked up as I applied fresh makeup. I started the car and flipped on the radio, hoping some music would lift my spirits.

Ashanti's sweet, angelic voice rang in my ears. The song? "Always on Time."

A sign, perhaps? Maybe it means my period will be on time?

Only time would tell whether this was a reassuring sign from God or not. For the moment, I feared for Damien that my dad was going to find out about all of this and there would be a shotgun wedding on the horizon—except without the wedding part.

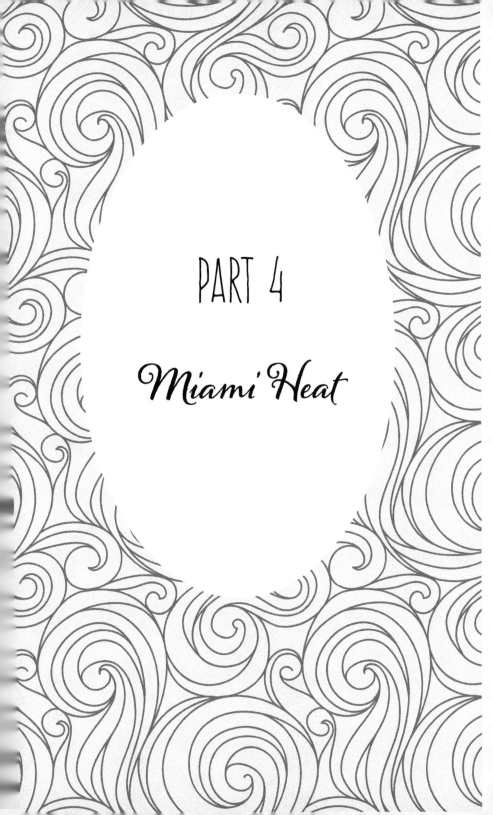

PART 4

Miami Heat

$\mathcal{T}$he scene: The bedroom of Karin's sorority house. This is set in the days pre-caller ID.

The phone rings.

Karin: Karin here.

Gina: Hey, it's me. What's good?

Karin: Hey, girl! Ya know, just livin' up the last two weeks of school.

Gina: What are you going to do once you graduate?

Karin: I don't know. I was hoping Damien would invite me to move to Queens with him.

Gina: If he hasn't asked you by now, it's not looking promising. I have an idea. Why not move to Coconut Grove and live with me? I need a roommate. I have plenty of space and you can find a dancing or acting gig here.

Karin: Really? That sounds *amazing*! I'd love to live in Miami. But...what about Damien?

Gina: I dunno. You'd do long distance, I guess.

Karin: Maybe.... Then again, I bet he'd follow me if I moved. If he doesn't, it'd be a sign that we're not meant to be—don't you think? There's probably lots of hot guys in Miami, anyway.

Gina: Yup—and rich ones, too. So—you in?

Karin: Hell, yeah! See you in Miami!

Gina: Awesome! You're gonna love it.

Karin: I'm so excited!

Gina: Me too! First thing when you get here—we're gonna get Brazilian bikini waxes! Bye!

Karin: Bye. *Wait...*

The phone clicks.

Karin: *...what?!!!*

End scene.

TWENTY-ONE

My Burning Bush

I WAS LUCKY ON TWO COUNTS: I DIDN'T END UP GETTING PREGNANT from Damien's super sperm; and, as I hoped, he trailed me to Florida. Unfortunately, as I'll soon reveal, I was slammed by more medical drama as the summer unfolded.

I paid rent by waiting tables at Houston's restaurant in Coral Gables. I didn't give up on my acting ambitions, however, taking acting classes on Saturdays.

During one lesson on character development, I felt an uncontrollable urge to pee. It was all too familiar. There was no denying my condition when I plopped down on the toilet and re-experienced that burning, tingling sensation.

"*Another UTI?! No friggin' way!*" V groaned.

Afraid that she was right, I looked into the bowl beneath me.

Oh no. Blood. And it's definitely not my period.

"*Told you so!*" V rubbed it in.

"But V...*there was no blood with the last UTI.*"

"*Uh-oh—time to abandon ship!*"

No matter the cause of our affliction, I had to grin and bear it for the remaining hour of my class.

I buckled up and rejoined my classmates to watch them perform their final scenes. I skipped the usual chitchat after class ended and sped off in my new two-week-old Mitsubishi Lancer.

I speed dialed Damien along the way. "Listen," I directed. "I need you to go to Publix and get Northland Cranberry Juice—the kind with twenty-seven percent cranberry juice—right away."

"Sure," he responded. "Is everything all right?"

"No, it's *not* all right," my voice cracked. "I have a fucking urinary tract infection and it's *bad*."

I regretted swearing at him, but I was on Interstate 95, doing 95 mph, and about to pee in my pants. Venting to someone was my only legitimate release.

As if my verbal assault on him wasn't enough, I nearly ran him over as I pulled into the driveway. When I leapt out of the car, I realized he was holding up a big glass of red juice for me.

My mind registered that he'd come through for me yet again, but I didn't have time to offer gratitude. I gulped down the liquid all at once and sprinted into the house to my obvious destination. A few moments later....

Seriously, V—only three drops? This is maddening! I feel like I'm holding back the Hoover Dam.

Uh, oh. More blood.

Now I really freaked out. This shouldn't be happening. I considered going to the hospital, but I couldn't afford the visit. What waitress has health insurance?

My natural inclination was to blame Damien: "You probably didn't wash your dick well enough or something."

"I washed it the same as always," he defended himself. "Don't blame me. Drink some more juice. You probably just need to pee out all of the infection."

"So, now you're a doctor?"

Then it hit me.

Gina's dad is a doctor. Why didn't I think of this sooner?

My roommate was busily freshening up after her daily run, but she came downstairs shortly after I summoned her. I filled her in on my symptoms and situation, and she didn't hesitate to call her father. As she described my ailment to him, I imagined Dr. Johnson nodding and saying the obligatory "Mn-hmns."

Then she shoved the phone at me.

This is weird. I know he's a doctor...but he's also my friend's father. What choice do I have?

I sucked it up and explained everything to him all over again.

"What do you think, Dr. Johnson?"

"I'll write a prescription for you that should take care of it," he replied.

Phew!

All of sudden, the awkwardness vanished. I pictured the doctor looking like Mekhi Phifer when he was on *ER* TV show.

This man is my hero!

"Our *hero!*" V corrected.

A moment later, Dr. Johnson asked an unusual question: "Are you allergic to sulfa?"

"Huh? Sulfur? I put sulfur on my—"

"No, *sulfa,*" he interrupted, "It's a type of antibiotic."

"Oh," I answered. "No, I don't think I'm allergic to that—just penicillin."

"Great," he decided. "I'm going to call in some Bactrim for you. You'll be feeling better in no time. If not, call me back."

"Thank you so much, Dr. Johnson, *thank you,*" I emphasized before we said our goodbyes.

Gina couldn't stop laughing at me. It wasn't intended to be mean; rather, it was a "You *would* get yourself into this kind of situation"-type laugh.

Since there was no way I could have made it to the drugstore and back without some kind of piss bucket under the driver's seat, I begged Damien to pick up the medicine for me.

I'm sure he hurried his mission as much as possible, but no amount of time would have satisfied me. When he returned, I whisked the prescription bag out of his hand like a drug addict desperate for her fix.

Soon V and I will be in the clear. I'll be feeling like a million bucks by morning.

As usual, the universe had other plans in store.

One of Gina's and my favorite pastimes was watching old episodes of *Sex in the City* on DVD while slurping Appleton rum and Coke. Fifteen minutes into the episode and halfway through my drink, my head started to itch.

Sip, scratch. Sip, scratch. Sip, scratch....

"Ugh," I said, digging my nails into my scalp. Nothing seemed to alleviate the sensation.

"What is it?" Gina asked.

"My head is really itchy," I twitched.

"Did you wash your hair today?" Gina chuckled.

"Yeah, I had to for the acting class," I answered.

I resituated myself on the couch to take my mind off my itchy head. My first thought went to....

Lice. How the hell could I have lice? Wait—the dog!

Gina had a greyhound rescue named Wilder. "Maybe Wilder has fleas?" I proposed.

"No way!" she protested. "Wait—did you say your head is itchy?"

"Yeah, it's weird," I considered, revealing portions of skin to her. "It's all around the nape of my neck and stuff."

"Oh no—look at your arms! Do you happen to have hives?"

I rolled up my sleeves and screeched in disgust: "Shit, I *do*! I'm covered!"

"You're allergic to the sulfa!" she confirmed.

"Am I going to die?" I asked myself, turning to her as if she were the doctor. "Like—is my throat going to close?"

"No," she said, sounding much like her father. "But I'd suggest you take some Benadryl right away."

I was a young adult working a summer waitressing job, so it wasn't like I had Benadryl packets or bottles strewn around my bedroom. My next move was pretty predictable.

"*Daaaaammmmmiiieeeeennn!*" I screamed upward.

He had been upstairs playing video games in order to protect his fragile brain from being subjected to a single frame of *Sex and the City*.

He clumped down the stairs in a panic. "What is it? What's wrong?" he asked.

"Look!" I exclaimed, thrusting my arms in front of his nose. The welts were expanding to the size of quarters by this point. "I've broken out all over! I'm allergic to the medicine."

"Damn!" he reacted.

"I need you to take me to CVS for some Benadryl—right now!"

"Okay—I'll get my keys."

The itch now permeated my body from head to toe. I scratched everywhere like a crazy person. My face looked puffed out and contorted like Will Smith's in the movie *Hitch*.

I don't even remember the drive to the drugstore, but I do recall racing through the aisles in a desperate search for Benadryl. I wasn't messing around with the store brand; this situation demanded the real stuff.

I was so embarrassed by my appearance that I coaxed Damien into bringing the medicine up to the register and paying for it. He shook his head the entire time between when the cashier rang it up to when I dragged him by his shirt through the parking lot to the parked car.

As he peeled out of the parking spot, I tore open the box and safety seal. I didn't bother checking the dosage, instead pouring the liquid into the plastic cup at a level that seemed right to me.

Down the hatch!

I swallowed the medicine back like a shot, licking the inside of the cup with my tongue to get every last drop.

"Ya sure you got it all?" Damien mocked.

We burst out laughing. "Thank goodness this wasn't our first date," I remarked.

"Yeah, it would've been our last," he joked. "You seriously need to pee every time after sex."

"I *did*—I swear!"

Long before we arrived at the house, I decided I'd had enough rum and Coke and *Sex and the City* for the day. The moment we entered I announced, "I'm going to lie down upstairs."

"I'm going to finish your drink, then," Damien countered. "I deserve it after all this."

"Go for it," I waved back at him.

I started to feel woozy halfway up the steps. I chalked it up to the combination of UTI, allergy, rum, sulfa, and Benadryl.

I collapsed on my futon bed and did my best imitation of a corpse. A while later, Damien presented me with a fresh glass of cranberry juice.

How sweet. He must have made another run to the supermarket for me. I didn't even have to ask. He's stepping up big-time. This guy is marriage material.

I chugged it down with one hand while continuing to scratch with the other. I squeezed his hand and uttered, "Thank you."

"No problem," he said, petting my head.

I hate when he does that. I feel like a dog.

"Wait," I called back to him. "Something is wrong."

I began to feel dizzy. The room pulsated in and out.

Afraid I'd pass out if I stood up by myself, I began crawling across the carpet like a sloth. "Help me up," I said. "I think I need to go to the bathroom again."

He dutifully supported my weight until we reached the bathroom. This time, I had a very different kind of urgent issue....

I shoved him out of the way, slamming the door on his nose and locking it. I flipped open the toilet lid open and lowered my face down to the bowl. A category 1 storm had been brewing inside me.

I retched violently, relieving my stomach of what felt like a year's worth of food and liquid.

During a brief lull, he asked through the door: "Are you okay?"

"Yes," I replied.

Splat!

"I'll be...fine."

Splat!

I feel like I'm going to die.

I was given enough of a reprieve to raise my head for a cleansing breath. I wiped my smeared mouth and cheeks with toilet paper. I couldn't help glance at the contents of the toilet bowl—lots of swirling red.

Of course, cranberry juice!

I flushed and leaned back, my eyes glued to the toilet. Nausea could resume at any moment.

"Do you want me to hold your hair?" Damien offered.

No, I don't want you to see me like this. My skin is covered in hives. I have vomit all over my face. My breath reeks. I'm sweating like a marathoner. Stay out there. Please. In fact, go away and don't come back until tomorrow.

"No—I'm good," I finally uttered.

I started to feel a little better: The stars disappeared; my breathing slowed; and my stomach stopped churning. I felt strong enough to get to my feet and step over to the sink, where I rinsed my mouth out with cold water.

I unlocked and opened the door and shot him a sad face with puppy dog eyes.

I hope that distracts him from how disgusting I sounded.

Damien assisted me back toward the bedroom, where he tucked me into the futon. He sat in my director's chair and regarded me with a look of concern.

Fifteen minutes later: *BAM!*

My face once again hovered over the toilet bowl. This time was even uglier than the first because there was less cranberry juice in my system to throw up. The dry heaves kicked in. Clearly, my body was rejecting the concoction I'd ingested. I thought it couldn't get any worse when....

Oh no, no, no, no!

My bowels rumbled like Mount Vesuvius.

Please, God, not diarrhea, too! I can't handle this.

I was far less concerned about my medical condition than I was about subjecting Damien to my ordeal. Even though we'd been dating for four years, it was too soon into living together. There was no ring, no vows of for better or worse. He could bail at the first sight (or smell) of the squirts!

I flipped around for the impending eruptions. The stomach cramps were excruciating. I remained there for some time waiting to see if another bout would hit. In my haste, I noticed I hadn't managed to lock the door.

Damien barged in to find me sitting on the toilet shooting him a death glare.

You can't see me like this!

The barnyard stench was so overwhelming that, try as he might, he couldn't conceal his wrinkling nostrils and furrowed eyebrows.

"I'm shitting my brains out—close the door! Leave!" I shrieked.

"Sorry," he mewled, the door barreling shut.

Once able to pull myself together, I sheepishly opened the door.

He'd been waiting for me with the expression of a guilty child who had received a scolding.

"Well," I began, "we crossed a new boundary today."

"We did. But I still love you," he said, once again patting the top of my head. "Go lie down and rest."

I dragged myself toward the bedroom with what little dignity I had left. Along the way I was well aware of him reaching his hand into the bathroom to turn on the fan in an attempt to air out the space.

All of this, thanks to a little bacteria in my vagina!

One thing I realized: If he could make it through this ordeal with me, he would stand by me through anything....

TWENTY-TWO

Getting Buzzed

SOME GUYS MAY WONDER WHAT WAITRESSES TALK ABOUT WHEN they are trying to pass the time doing side work—the job they are assigned each night in a restaurant after closing. (This usually consists of things such as cleaning the coffee machine, polishing silverware, or stacking the glassware.)

Easy answer: They discuss the same thing as the waiters: *sex*.

One night, the subject somehow came around to vibrators. I was intrigued because I had never used or owned such a device. Even if I'd had one, I probably would have used it incorrectly and short-circuited the power grid.

Back in those days, you couldn't flick on your computer and browse online in private mode in the comfort of your own home to select the perfectly crafted model and have it shipped to you in a (hopefully) nondescript box. If you wanted a vibrator, you had to summon up enough courage to physically enter one of those creepy adult bookstores or an even seedier sex shop.

"I just bought a brand new, deluxe, high-powered vibrator," Jada boasted while straightening up the liquor bottles in the service bar. It sounded to me like she was describing a Hoover vacuum cleaner. "I got off three times yesterday."

I was shocked that Jada was being so open. She was a young Black student at Miami University and came from a wealthy military background. She was the last person I expected to be masturbating (or at least admit to it so candidly).

"At one time or three separate times?" Carissa probed as she walked by with a stack of glassware. By contrast, she was a blonde bombshell who always earned huge tips and was in an on-again-off-again relationship with one of the bartenders.

"Yeah, at once—it was mind-blowing!" Jada exclaimed. "How many times a day do you masturbate?"

"Depends on how bored I am," Carissa considered. "My record is six."

"Where'd you get your vibrator?" Paulina asked. "I need something stronger and more intense."

Holy crap, does everyone diddle themselves except me?

Jada referenced a place called Pleasure Emporium, which sounded like a whole other tube of lube. She described it as a BJ's warehouse of sexual paraphernalia, with aisle after aisle of amazing toys and gizmos. Several of the waitresses then proudly admitted to being customers of the establishment. Someone chimed in with a joke that the Emporium should offer their own rewards program. I started to feel like the odd girl out, like I was missing some secret social scene.

"What about you, Freeland? How many times a day do you masturbate?" Paulina pressed.

Shit—what do I say? I don't own a vibrator. If I lie and they ask me questions, they'll see right through me.

"Oh, you know, that's not really my thing," I hedged. "Damien is *so good* that I don't need one."

All things considered, I thought I'd given them a darn good answer. Instead of nodding and moving on, however, they burst into laughter.

"You don't know what you're missing!" Jada howled. "How can you not? It's *sooooo amazing*. When you place that vibrator up to your clit and feel the power surging between your legs…it just…it becomes lit up, your head rolls back, your pussy pulses uncontrollably…. No guy can do that, I don't give a shit what kind of magician he is."

My face burned crimson from embarrassment.

The general manager entered the room just in the nick of time, saving me from further embarrassment. "Ladies, come on," he urged us. "Less talk, more work. Let's get out of here before 1:00 AM tonight."

It ended the conversation—for now. Yet no matter how hard I tried I couldn't get Jada's multiorgasmic image out of my head.

I also had to contend with V's prodding. *"Pleasure Emporium— what are we waiting for? Maybe they're open 24/7. Come on, let's go!"*

"I am not going into a place like that. It's…sleazy."

"Sounds like everyone is having a party except us," V whined. *"I never get to have any fun. I want some of that power surging, pulsating action!"*

"No way," I argued. *"Someone might recognize me."*

That seemed to settle things, at least until the following weekend when a couple of my sorority sisters—Jeanine and Nora—came to visit. I was elated at the prospect of showing them around town and helping them enjoy the best time ever.

Of course, South Beach was number one on our list. We went to all of the usual cool hangouts: Wet Willies, Clevelander's, and Mango's. Suffice it to say, I ingested more than my share of beers as we hopped from place to place. Along the way, I had just enough consciousness to spot a certain storefront, the news of which rapidly traveled to V.

"There it is! It's right over there—Pleasure Emporium! Let's check it out!" V encouraged.

"Behave yourself," I berated her.

My friends and I entered a nearby bar, where we sat at a table and downed a few more beers while recounting the day's adventures and gaping at the shirtless, muscular guys hovering around the outdoor area.

"I don't ever want to leave this town," Jeanine professed. "You're so lucky you get to live here, Z."

"I'm definitely not complaining!" I agreed.

"I need a cold shower after all this action and testosterone," Nora fanned herself.

"Yeah, we should probably get out of here before I assault one of them," Jeanine added.

We laughed, polished off the remainder of beer in our glasses, and stood up. Correction...my *friends* were on their feet. I stumbled.

I was in the worst shape among our trio, though none of us was fit to drive. Not that they could have handled my car anyway, since I drove a stick shift. "Maybe we should...walk around for a little bit before we get in the car?" I suggested.

"Yeah, good idea," Nora said as we made our way to the exit.

"Where should we go?" Jeanine asked as we stepped onto the street and looked around.

It was still broad daylight, but a certain neon sign glowed right at me: "PLEASURE EMPORIUM."

"What are we waiting for? It's playtime!" V roared.

The gallons of beer and V's pressure had weakened my resolve. Not to mention that I was more than a bit curious.

It's better than drunk driving, isn't it?

"Actually," I sheepishly began, "there is one store I've been meaning to check out...it happens to be right across the street."

"*That* place?" Jeanine gestured. "Are you crazy?"

"Why not?" I asked. "It'll be fun! I heard everyone in Miami goes there."

Did I really just say that? What is the matter with me?

"Maybe they have some clothes?" Nora asked, scrambling to keep up the pace. "I could really use a cover-up to go over my bathing suit."

"Um," I considered. Now I was apparently the sex shop authority. "I doubt they offer much in the way of things that will cover you up."

We marched up to the building and glared at the door. My friends paused, visibly experiencing second thoughts.

"What the fuck, Karin?" Jeanine hesitated. "This seems crazy, even by our drunken standards."

"Yeah, I don't know if I can do it," Nora demurred.

"Oh, come on, don't be pussies," I railed at them.

Wait a minute. How did I suddenly become the one pressuring the others to do this? I feel like I'm hazing them.

"Don't worry, it'll be fine. We'll stick together the whole time," I promised.

"All right, I'm down," Nora consented. "I'm curious to see what they have in there. Besides, I really do need that cover-up."

It was two against one, which was good enough for me. At this point, Jeanine would have to follow me inside or stand alone in the blistering Florida sun.

As I pulled open the front door with authority, I felt the anxious presence of both friends hiding behind me. To my astonishment, we were met by two *greeters*. No, not the octogenarians you might find at a Walmart. These tattooed women in skimpy black leather outfits were around my age and had an assortment of jewelry on and in all parts of their faces—ears, noses, eyebrows, lips, and tongues.

"Welcome to Pleasure Emporium!" they sang, beaming from ear to ear. "Let us know if you need anything special."

They were probably the best professional greeters I'd ever seen. Not only that, the place smelled like someone was baking sugar cookies. The customers weren't sketchy at all. In fact, they all seemed like regular, upstanding citizens.

We perused up and down the aisles, not expecting to buy anything. I, for one, believed I was there for curiosity purposes and perhaps a laugh or two. We broke out into hysterics at the sight of the ridiculous dildos of every size, color, and shape on the shelves. I resisted the temptation to touch and squeeze one. I don't know why, but I imagined the texture would be like stress balls—only shaped like the other male genitalia.

Meanwhile, V was in her sexual Disney World. *"I want that one! No, THAT one!"*

I ignored her and pressed on, grabbing my friends' hands. This shopping excursion with my girlfriends was turning out to be a real hoot!

Sure enough, they did have *some* clothes—but I doubted the titty tassels were going to fill Nora's need. We realized it was a fool's mission when we turned a corner into the whips and chains aisle. Each of us grabbed a different whip, so we could feign whacking each other. We made goofy noises of pleasure and pain, but really it all came out as girlish snickering.

We must look like such assholes.

We pressed on, eventually becoming comfortable enough to part ways and browse independently. Nothing grabbed my attention, until...I heard a strange buzzing sound.

Suddenly, I felt all eyes upon me. I tried not to engage anyone, instead pretending that I was considering an item on the shelf.

The buzzing drew nearer.

V's radar turned up, like a bat with sonar. *"Oooh, I wonder what that is...."*

A moment later, one of the greeters from the front of the store stood right in my grill; she waved an object at me. Try as I might to avert my eyes, I could not look away—especially since she danced the object just inches away. The pink vibrator in her hand was like a magic wand. It resembled a plastic utensil in Barbie's kitchen. The instrument was about four inches long, an inch in diameter, and had an on-off switch on the side and featured two speeds: cruise control and turbo.

"Feel this," she offered.

I giggled and dumbly alternated between staring at her and the vibrator.

I wonder how she ended up working in a store like this. Did she respond to an ad? What qualifications were required? What kind of questions did she have to answer during the interview (assuming there was one)?

"See how powerful it is," she teased, taking the liberty of grabbing my hand and bringing it toward the vibrator. My hand jerked back—a reflex.

"Come on, just give it a *feel*," she persisted. "It's a *really good one*. You won't be sorry."

What a fantastic greeter/salesperson! She should get a raise!

She reclaimed my hand, this time drawing the tip of my pointer finger to the edge of the vibrator. It gently tickled my skin.

"OH MY GOD!" V swooned. "*We need that, STAT!*"

I had to admit I was intrigued! The saleswoman/greeter knew she had me exactly where she wanted me. She launched into a demonstration—well, not an actual demonstration on her lady parts, but one that enabled me to understand the features of the device and how it operated. I came to find out it was a clitoral vibrator, intended for external stimulation only.

Thank goodness—I am not sticking anything in V other than a tampon and Damien.

She pointed out how it came with a removable cap, on which were pointy little plastic protrusions.

I wonder if those hurt....

Under the cap were four metal rounded bumps. She showed me how to turn the vibrator on and off and how easy it was to change the batteries. "Not only will this get you to paradise and back, the batteries are included," she upsold. (I had no idea how valuable free batteries were going to be.)

What a deal!

I had no clue whether this was the Volkswagen or Jaguar of vibrators. It was pink and it vibrated. What else should I have been looking for in a vibrator? I wondered what questions I should have asked....

Do you have to wait thirty minutes after eating? Would it electrocute me in the shower? Is there a time restriction—like how you're only supposed to sit in a hot tub for fifteen minutes?

Hypnotized, I trailed after the young woman to the front counter right in front of my sorority sisters. They couldn't believe what they were seeing. I refused to bat an eyelash, which would have given away that this was completely out of character for me.

"How much is it?" I asked, opening up my purse.

At this point, money was no object. I would have spent fifty dollars, if it cost that much. There was no backing down.

"Nineteen ninety-nine," she answered.

What a bargain!

I imagined the absurdity of having to come back to exchange or return the device, should it be defective. "Does this come with a ninety-day money-back satisfaction guarantee or a warranty?"

"All vibrator sales are final—but don't worry. I have this one at home and, believe me, you'll be satisfied."

As she processed my credit card, I wondered if she was going to put it in a big bag with the Pleasure Emporium name and logo on the side. My purse was too small to fit the vibrator inside of it, and I didn't want to be a walking advertisement for this place.

Fortunately, she plunked my new buddy in a white opaque paper bag along with the receipt.

I collected my friends and strutted out. Although they'd wimped out on making any purchases, they had no qualms about pestering me to check out what was in my white opaque bag. I flashed it open to show them the goods.

"*Holy shit!*" they gaped in awe. "*You really bought it!*"

Enough time had elapsed that I was sober and fine to drive.

I arrived home to find Damien fast asleep in our bedroom. He had to work late that night, so he was grabbing a nap before his shift.

This was something of a blessing because I had zero intention of telling Damien about my purchase or where my friends and I had been. I tucked the bag away at the bottom of my drawer for the time being.

This is my little secret.

"*No, it isn't,*" V corrected. "*It's OUR little secret.*"

TWENTY-THREE

Bare Beaver

V and I waited patiently for just the right private moment to become acquainted with the new purchase. Everything had to be perfect for our first time. Who knew I was such a hopeless romantic?

Meanwhile, I had been procrastinating on getting a bikini wax. Gina wouldn't stop nagging me about it. I knew I couldn't put her off forever, but the idea of having hot wax spread on my pubic hair and then yanked apart from the follicles did not strike me as a pleasant way to spend a morning.

Then it occurred to me that a smooth, freshly mowed lady garden might be the ideal way to introduce V to my vibrator. I also had a feeling Damien would appreciate the new look and a clear runway down there.

I gave the "all systems go" sign to Gina, who set up an appointment for me with European Wax Center because word had it that their wax was "gentler." We scheduled it for two weeks out so the hair could grow to an acceptable length—even though I didn't know those specific measurements—and to steel myself for the dreaded day.

The appointment was to occur first thing on a Saturday morning. This had the benefit of my body being scoured enough for a stranger to enter my jungle. By this point, *jungle* was an understatement. I couldn't even wear shorts in public because the hair crept so far down my thighs.

I admit I do not have a high tolerance for pain. As I sat in the waiting room and faked reading a women's magazine until it was my turn to be called, I sweated like a pig. I trembled so much I wondered how I was one day going to handle childbirth.

A gorgeous Indian woman in her early twenties with full makeup and expertly manicured nails shouted out my name as if I were running for office: "*Karin Freeland!*"

Ugh—why couldn't I have gotten some old grandma instead? She is totally going to judge V and me.

The waxer led me down the hall.

"My name is Priya," she introduced herself. "We're in room four today. Everything from the waist down off."

Once in the private room, she rolled out a fresh piece of tissue paper across what seemed to be a massage table. She gave the hot purple wax on the counter a stir and then promptly exited, closing the door behind her.

That's it? No chitchat? You're about to look at my vagina! I need to be courted. Perhaps I should tell her I'm a bikini wax virgin?

And…where is the cover for my lower body? They even give me one at the gynecologist!

Time was ticking. I didn't want to be caught disrobing, so I swiftly removed my jean skirt and thong.

Hmn…do I leave my sneakers on? It's kinda weird to be half-naked except for footwear. I guess I should take them off, too.

Naked and uncomfortable, I sat on the table with my hands covering my goods and listened to the pop music blasting over the speakers until the waxer finally reentered the room.

"Okay, let's see what we're working with," she said in a clinical voice.

After a cursory examination she muttered, "Not bad. How do you want it?"

"I've never had one before," I admitted. "What…are the options?"

"Well, you can go bare—or you can leave a little landing strip."

I figured the latter would be less painful and not make me look like a ten-year-old down there. I wanted some remaining semblance of my womanhood. "Okay, let's go with landing strip."

She came at me with a pair of shiny scissors. They may as well have been hedge clippers. V tightened closed.

She sensed my nerves and tried to calm me. "It's okay, you'll be fine," she comforted. "I just need to trim the hair first to make it easier to wax. Relax and spread your legs."

That last sentence with the contradictory words "relax" and "spread your legs" could not possibly have been more intimidating.

How can a woman relax while spreading her legs for a complete stranger? Wait. Maybe I should ask for her credentials before she starts on this procedure? I mean…I hope this isn't her first week on the job.

I did everything *except* relax. My teeth clenched. My nails dug through the tissue paper and into the table. Despite my reactions, she went about her businesses slathering wax on me. It was definitely hot but, thankfully, not enough to burn. The purple, odorless goo was thicker than other waxes I'd used on my eyebrows and facial hair.

She waited the seemingly requisite amount of time for the wax to cool and perform its adhesive magic. As if an alarm had sounded in her head, Priya began her countdown: "Ready. Here we go: *one, two….*"

Zzzzzrriiitttt!

Off came one strip like separating Velcro.

Hey! Ouch! Whatever happened to three?!

Zzzzzrriiitttt!

Off came the second trip.

Yow! I'm an idiot for letting Gina pressure me into this. It was a terrible idea. What are those Brazilian women thinking? You can keep your waxing—I don't want any part of this!

She repeated my punishment a few more times until I presumed we were finished.

Zzzzzrriiitttt! Zzzzzrriiitttt! Zzzzzrriiitttt!

But no. She had plenty more torture in store for me.

"Flip over," Priya ordered.

"What's that?" I questioned. "Sounded like you said, 'flip over.'"

"Yeah," she replied. "I have to get your rear."

Not only had I felt I'd endured more than enough pain and suffering, I wasn't about to be surcharged for something I didn't need. "Is that really part of it? Is it…necessary?"

"Yes, it's part of it—and you should get it."

"Oh," I abjectly accepted.

I tried to hide my embarrassment as I rolled over on all fours. She went into the same routine, spreading hot wax on my crack…

How humiliating….

Once again, she waited for the wax to cool, counted to two, and then let it rip.

Zzzzzrriiitttt!

Yow!

Zzzzzrriiitttt!

Yow!

Zzzzzrriiitttt!

Yow! Will this torture ever end?

And then, miraculously, it did.

"You're all set—looking brand new!" she announced like an obstetrician having delivered a baby girl.

I didn't share her enthusiasm, though. I paid and zipped out of there as if she was going to splash wax all over the rest of me. On the drive home, I started to notice something about my nether regions….

Smooth…this feels nice…maybe it wasn't such a bad idea after all.

I often wondered how women could go through the agony of childbirth and then do it all over again with a second child. I was starting to understand: The reward must be so great it eliminates all memory of the pain and suffering.

In my case, I now had complete amnesia of my traumatic

experience. I became overjoyed at the prospect of unveiling my new 'do to Damien.

When I arrived at our apartment, he was still asleep in bed with the blinds shielding the room from sunshine. I wasted no time sliding off my underwear and climbing into bed with my skirt still on.

"Hey—wake up," I poked him, nuzzling my face into his chest while my hand traveled south down his body. I wanted him to know exactly what I was up to.

"Come on, I'm exhausted, Karin," he protested.

"I know, but I want to show you something *special*," I leered, guiding his hand between my legs. When he didn't respond, I added, "I just had a Brazilian wax."

That was all the incentive he needed. In an instant he positioned me on top of him. "Whoa there, cowboy," I giggled.

His eyes widened as he took a peek under my skirt. "This is even hotter than I'd imagined," he gaped.

Giddyap! Everyone is a satisfied customer: Damien, V, and me.

TWENTY-FOUR

Good Vibrations

A FEW DAYS PASSED AND V WAS STILL AS SMOOTH AS A HAIRLESS cat. At long last, I was able to set up a private date to break in my virgin vibrator. I figured out the perfect day and time with the least chance of interruption: Thursday evening. Damien had a closing shift, which meant he wouldn't arrive home before 3:00 AM. That left plenty of time for my sexcapade.

I sat on the couch and watched TV while Damien prepared himself for work. My right foot tapped with anticipation.

When Damien emerged, he asked, "So, what are you going to do tonight?"

Like anyone who is up to no good, I felt paranoid.

He knows! My body language on the couch is giving me away! Or… maybe he found the vibrator?

"I don't know," I innocently responded. "I'll probably just paint my nails and watch some reruns."

"Okay, have fun!" he said, planting a farewell kiss on my cheek.

He seemed to take forever to leave. He took one last bathroom break, searched around for his keys, fumbled around for cigarettes….

Why won't he just get out of here already? I have a date!

He stepped out the door. I watched him through the window as he plodded from the courtyard to the parking lot. I tiptoed into our bedroom in order to best hear his Honda CRX exit the gate. A familiar-sounding engine turned on before the sounds of Outkast blasted through his partially open window. He backed out, swerved around, and zoomed through the gate.

Finally—alone!

I shot back to the door to double-check that it was locked; not just the deadbolt but the chain, too. I wasn't going to take any chances.

I'm like a kid lighting up a joint for the first time while my parents are away....

I skipped to my bedroom and opened the drawer where I'd hid my toy. I rummaged through several pairs of socks before finding the familiar white bag.

I attempted to tear through the packaging like an overly zealous child opening a birthday gift. Just one problem: The packaging was plastic, and I needed something to cut through it. I dashed to the kitchen and found some scissors in a drawer.

Is all of this protection really necessary? Was the vibrator really going to break out of the packaging?

I couldn't wait to start playing with it (or, more precisely, *it* with *me*). My heart raced. V became gushing wet.

Why are we already so hot?

Despite being anxious, I took a moment to read the instructions. I suppose I didn't want to risk any unnecessary, embarrassing injuries that I wouldn't be able to explain to Damien or a hospital nurse.

The directions seemed pretty simple. Slide open the compartment, insert two double A batteries—positive and negative facing the right way—and then seal it back up. All I had to do now was flip the *on* switch—except I hesitated.

I've never done this before. It seems crude to just turn it on and "go." Don't I need a drink first? Some lit candles and soft mood music? A little romantic small talk? Lights on or off?

I left the lights off as I continued to debate the process in my head.

"Let's get this show on the road, girl!" V hollered. "Take off your shorts and underwear and get in bed already!"

I removed my shorts and panties and lay down on the bed, tugging the sheets over my entire body. I wanted to be completely hidden from the outside world...and anyone up in heaven—like my grandparents—who might be looking down on me with disapproval.

Here goes nothing....

I slid my finger across the *on* button. The vibrator buzzed like a power saw. It was a lot louder than I recalled from the demo at the store.

Crap—my next-door neighbors are going to complain about this racket. I flicked it off.

I tiptoed into my closet. I removed a few shirts from their hangers, stuffing them in front of the vent to block the sound from getting through to my neighbors.

I returned to bed, gearing up for another attempt. I flipped the vibrator back on and lowered it to my clit. The sensations sizzled throughout my entire body.

Wow, this is amazing—and I'm only on cruise control! I can do this all day long.

I was unsure of what to do next.

"Why don't you try moving it around a little?" V suggested.

I gingerly maneuvered it: a little on the sides, back to the middle, come up under the hood. I needed to position it in just the right spot.

I know it's there...somewhere.

My head became foggy. My hearing muffled from the blood rushing to my head.

I'm getting closer...closer...

BAM!

I became dismayed when my clitoris began to feel numb. Then I remembered that the plastic cover adorning the vibrator was removable.

I flipped off the cap. It rolled down between my butt cheeks. *Great...*

I fished it out and tossed it aside. I went back to concentrating on the task at hand, pressing the metallic bumps against my clit. They felt cold down there, so I backed off a bit. I gradually eased the softness of the rounded tip against me. This was even more intense than before, reawakening my somewhat numbed senses.

"This is more like it!" V raved. *"That bikini wax was a pretty good idea after all."*

"Shhh, V," I cautioned. *"You're spoiling the moment."*

I rubbed it against myself more vigorously. My nerves turned ablaze. My feet began to tingle. A rush made its way up my legs, through V, and into my stomach, where a million butterflies flitted about.

"This is it!" V exclaimed. *"Don't stop whatever it is you're doing!"*

The rush didn't stop. It roamed through my chest, making my nipples stand at attention before advancing through my neck to my face and ears. I squeezed my eyes shut.

Is this truly going to be the moment V and I have been waiting for?

I clutched the vibrator as tightly as I could to my clit until there was nowhere else for it to go.

Yes, yes, yes! This is it!

V quivered with uncontrollable undulation. My head arched until my back floated above the bed. I forgot all about my neighbors. Nor did I care if Damien barreled through the front door. I lost control over my vocal cords.

Uuuughhhh!!!

Then: an avalanche of relief and utter relaxation. Twenty-two years of stress melted out of my body. I collapsed, motionless. Even V remained atypically speechless.

I could barely comprehend what had just happened. I became aware of the vibrator continuing to buzz in my hand.

I don't want this feeling to end...ever!

As I basked in my post-euphoria, I used my index finger to turn off the vibrator. The room became eerily silent. I felt my clit with my left hand; it was still sensitive to the touch. I held it for just a moment.

Well—hello, clitoral orgasm! Nice to meet you—where have you been all my life?

I'm not defective after all. My body does work. Apparently, I can have an orgasm…only, it's with a machine.

I was then struck by mixed emotions.

I enjoy having sex with Damien. Why doesn't this ever happen when I'm with him? Why do I feel like I'm being unfaithful to him?

My head popped out from underneath the sheets. The fresh air felt good on my face. The corners of my lips curved upward into a wide smile.

Who is this expression for? I don't care—I just had my first Big O!

I wondered what my post-orgasm protocol should be.

Pee? Shower? The last thing I need is a UTI.

I made up my own ritual: pee, shower, and make the bed. Although Damien wasn't expected for hours, I didn't want to take the chance that he might show up early, see messy sheets, and wonder what I'd been doing under the covers. When I raised the sheets and blanket, something went flying.

What the hell is that? Oh, shit—the cap! Don't want Damien finding that.

I recovered it and brought it into the bathroom. I lathered the cap with soap and water before placing it back in my secret hide-away, along with the vibrator.

Mission accomplished.

"I feel like a new woman," V gushed.

"Yeah, you and me both!"

The rest of the evening returned to its regular programming. I sank back into the living room cushion with the remote and flipped channels. I had no idea what I was watching and didn't care.

My life is complete. At twenty-two, I've experienced my first mind-blowing, rip my hair out kinda orgasm. I had no idea it was possible for anything to feel this good. Time to commemorate the achievement.

I lit up a Kool cigarette, inhaled, and plotted my next date with my pink pal.

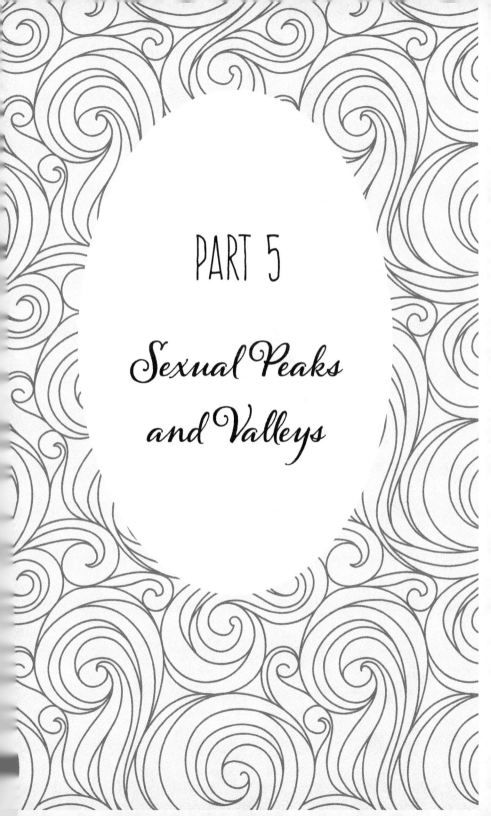

PART 5

Sexual Peaks and Valleys

THINGS THAT DON'T SUCK ABOUT GETTING OLDER

1. Getting a break on your car insurance at twenty-five.
2. Being brave enough to order a copy of the *Kama Sutra*.
3. Having enough money to pay for entertainment and fashion needs.
4. You can buy a pet.
5. Laughing when one of us gets sick instead of being embarrassed. ("I told you not to eat the rooster!")
6. Taking Caribbean vacations.
7. Having enough money to invest in high-class lingerie.
8. Being able to afford doctors and medication.
9. You can finally rent a hotel room.
10. Women enter their sexual peak.

THINGS THAT SUCK ABOUT GETTING OLDER

1. Hair in the wrong places: nose hair, chin hair, back hair… basically all body hair!
2. Sexual positions get stale and predictable. (How many times can it start in missionary?)
3. Work responsibilities take over free time.

4. You can't daydream about sex during a business meeting without being called on.
5. Your building super can hear you and your partner having sex in your tiny apartment.
6. You *need* to invest in lingerie to spice up your relationship.
7. It takes three days to recover from getting drunk instead of instant relief from a double bacon cheeseburger.
8. Men exit their sexual peak.
9. Exhaustion from just waking up in the morning.
10. IBS.
11. Bunions.
12. Sciatica.
13. Headaches.
14. Taxes.
15. General aches and pains with no identifiable cause.
16. Being too tired to have sex.

The obvious upshot of the above lists? Getting older *totally* sucks.

TWENTY-FIVE

The Ring of Fire

MIAMI WAS A BLAST, BUT DAMIEN AND I HAD TO GROW UP SOMETIME and move on with our lives and careers. He missed his family in New York, so it made sense for us to try our luck in the Big Apple. After all, what better place for me to pursue my acting career? We signed a lease for an apartment in Queens and I was fortunate enough to transfer with Houston's and secure a job right away.

Although our relationship remained strong, we found ourselves in different places, sexually speaking. I know, things tend to stop being so hot and heavy when couples are together for a lengthy period of time. I wondered whether he was exiting his sexual peak at the same time I was entering mine. Just my luck! The slack was filled by my newest best friend—the vibrator. Was the machine taking some of the sexual charge out of our relationship?

The vibrator became habitual and never failed to disappoint. In the morning before work: *check*. Happy hour: *check*. After dinner when Damien left the house: *check*.

The two of us made so much time, in fact, that I broke it! Why didn't I ask about paying extra for a long-term warranty?

This is a disaster! What am I going to do?

"You mean 'what are WE going to do?!'" V interjected.

In the days that passed, I realized how dependent V and I had become upon the vibrator. I wondered at what point such reliance tips over to being considered an addiction. Was I a sex addict?

I shrugged off my concerns, rationalizing my activity. Being orgasmless made me feel defective, lost, and bitchy, which was an intolerable situation. Since to my knowledge there was no such thing as a "vibrator repair shop" and I couldn't justify flying all the way back to Miami for a return visit to Pleasure Emporium, I went online to hunt down the perfect replacement toy.

Of course, in order to avoid any suspicion and distractions, I waited until Damien was at work to search for a site that seemed safe. I chose a seemingly reputable one (which, in retrospect, it most certainly was not; they asked for my Social Security number) and started browsing the goods to find something similar to my ole reliable pink pal. Unfortunately, the exact make and model didn't seem to exist anymore, and I had to settle for a smaller version fittingly called the Pocket Rocket. The upside was that this one could be used in the shower. *Sold!* I added it to the basket and clicked to the checkout screen.

I was about to seal the deal when I discovered that, for just a few dollars more, I could get free shipping. A few more seconds scrolling up and down led to spotting a few recommendations similar to my selected item. One, in particular, caught my eye....

Cock rings! It might be nice for Damien to wear something like that. Maybe it would get me closer to Orgasmville with him?

One of the cock rings even came assembled with a mini-vibrator—a two-for-one! What a deal! Not knowing which one would work better, I added both of them to my cart.

More items flashed on my screen. My endorphins flowed freely.

A butterfly-shaped vibrator with straps—how does that work? Oh. You wear it while you're having sex. I don't know if I'm ready for that yet, but it's pretty cheap—only fourteen ninety-nine, what a bargain!—so I better get that, too.

When the damage was done, not only did I earn free shipping, I spent so much that I earned a surprise free gift, too. What a delightful shopping experience!

In the coming days, I fretted over how my online pleasure treasure was going to be delivered. I prayed that the box wouldn't have the company name plastered all over it and that Damien wouldn't see it first and perhaps open it out of curiosity.

My bundles of joy arrived seven days later, boxed in nondescript white packaging. Unfortunately, Damien was home for its arrival and had to sign for it.

"Karin, you got a package!" he called from the front door.

I blasted through our apartment, knowing exactly what it was.

"Don't open that!" I exclaimed, realizing my reaction would make him even more suspicious.

"I wasn't going to," he said, tossing the box to me.

I was surprised that it felt so light. I imagined they protected the items inside really well with tissue paper or bubble wrap. I slinked toward the bedroom.

Damien's curiosity got the better of him "What's in the box?" he asked. "Aren't you going to open it?"

I shuddered.

This could be really embarrassing. Or damaging to our relationship. Maybe both.

"Just girl stuff, don't worry about it."

I should have known my answer wouldn't fly. We didn't hide anything from each other. "We've lived together for over two years now. I know about all your 'girl stuff.' It doesn't bother me. Just open it," he implored.

Ha! You don't know about ALL of my girl stuff.

"Eh, I'll do it later," I dismissed.

My attempt to play it cool and have him ignore the box was having the opposite effect. If anything, he was starting to become irritated. "Come on already, what's in there that you don't want me to see?"

The jig is up. I surrender.

"Fine," I huffed. "It's something for *both* of us—but, honestly, I don't know how you're going to feel about it."

I tore into the box with my nails, not even bothering to hunt down a knife or scissors.

"Maybe you should sit down for this," I suggested.

The tape peeled back and the flaps folded over. I felt inside through the tissue paper, grabbed hold of the first object, and presented it for both of us to see.

"What the fuck is that?!" he howled.

It took a couple of seconds for me to figure it out. I rotated it and looked at it from a few angles. It was bizarre, to say the least.

Oh, the butterfly vibrator!

"*Flap your wings over here, baby,*" V purred.

I cleared my throat to offer him my clinical explanation: "Well, Damien, this is a battery-operated device that I can wear during sex. The intent is to increase stimulation on my clitoris."

He looks befuddled. Maybe I'm being too clinical.

"I think it could be fun," I added.

He folded his arms. I should have predicted he would feel threatened. Most men probably would at the sight of this gadget. (And, in the reverse, if he had ordered a blow-up doll or pocket pussy, I would have done way more than crossed my arms.) "I don't get why you need it."

Once again, I dug my hand into the box of goodies. I studied the object and leapt with joy, hoping this new approach would win him over. "Oh, look! This one is for *you*! I mean, you wear it."

He stared at me with disapproval, his arms still folded.

"It's a cock ring with a mini-vibrator on it. I think you'll like how it feels!"

"It's *pink*, Karin!" he protested.

"I guess it is," I considered. "I think it takes a real man to wear pink."

"Don't give me that shit—I know about being a real man. Anyway, I thought you said it was a gift for *me*," he countered. "Hey, wait—where did you get this idea? *Cosmo*? The magazine that suggested guys might like a finger in the butt? Cuz this guy *doesn't*! You've got to stop reading that crap!"

"No, I didn't read it in *Cosmo*," I giggled, hoping to lighten the situation. "My old vibrator broke and I needed a new one—"

"*Old* vibrator?" he interrupted.

Busted! The cat is out of the bag.

"Yeah, I had one but—"

"And you never told me?"

"I didn't want you to become mad or jealous, like you're acting right now," I defended myself. "You know I can't have orgasms, and I just thought it might help."

"Well? Did it work?"

I lowered my head before softly delivering the blow: "Yes...."

"Well, *great*," he spat, turning away from me. "Then go off by yourself and enjoy your toys."

"Wait," I said, chasing after him. I grabbed his face with both hands and looked him in the eyes. "You don't understand. You get off every time we have sex. I want to enjoy it the way you do. I thought my body was broken, and I needed a way to find out if it was or wasn't. These devices are crazy powerful; there is no way you can replicate this. But that's why I bought some stuff for us to use *together*. I thought it would be something new and exciting for us. Please...can we just give them a try?"

I took a half-step back to give him room to soak it all in. I couldn't help but notice how hot he looked in his jeans and fresh white tee-shirt with that rough expression on his face. I was ready to strap on the butterfly and jump his bones right then and there.

Well...why not?

I couldn't afford to give him a chance to open his mouth and ruin my mood. I plunged my fingers into the box once more, this time extracting the Pocket Rocket. "Come on, I'll let you take *full control!*"

The corners of his mouth curled up into an involuntary grin.

I hooked him!

"Fine," he caved. "But no pink cock rings. Understood?"

"Deal."

"Do we need a safe word?" he questioned, sweeping me off my feet and into the bedroom.

"Um, no, I don't think that's going to be necessary."

Clearly, I have a lot to teach him—this is going to be a jam-packed night!

While the evening's romp was indeed educational and intensely pleasurable, something unexpected happened that I didn't fully understand at the time. The pressure to perform became more than I could take. Despite efforts that would have made the ancient Greeks blush, V and my head just wouldn't cooperate. If I had been alone, I would already have been satisfied three times over. In the end, when he asked if I'd orgasmed, I just didn't have the heart to lie, even though that would have been easier. I fessed up. He deserved more. I deserved more.

The only bonus was that he became more determined than ever to get me off. (The "surprise gift" with my purchases turned out not to be a bonus at all, but a nasty, allegedly edible lube gel, which both of us refused to try.) He was willing to explore all kinds of creative things, including experimenting with a topical cream that was sup-posed to enhance the feeling and improve the climax. (No dice.) Eventually, he even gave the cock ring a shot. (Definitely, no dice.) Sure, it started out fine. Midway, he threw me off him in screaming agony. I guess the cock ring had cut off the circulation to his mem-ber. He became so desperate he yanked the ring off in one swift motion, tearing it in half. I felt like returning the broken parts to the website and demanding a refund with a harsh letter ("It couldn't contain my boyfriend's schlong!") but, of course, I never did.

Desperate times called for desperate measures. Now that I was a full-grown, independent woman, I decided to have a rare, intimate conversation with my mother about sex—though, as far as she knew, I was still a virgin.

To my surprise, my mom had no qualms revealing that she'd never had any problem whatsoever achieving orgasm during sex. It wasn't hereditary, after all. Damn it!

The quest didn't end there. I bought a book that I thought contained all kinds of tips and tricks. Instead, it turned out to be a book of orgasm poetry. It was ethereal, filled with intangible thoughts. While I hoped to "manifest the invisible delight" as it suggested, I ended up becoming more confused than ever.

Next, Damien and I became intrigued by a still photo guide to the *Kama Sutra*. If it worked for so many people in India for all of these centuries, maybe it would do the trick for us? The positions looked pretty amazing and we couldn't wait to test out the classics: Silkworm, Cat and Mouse Share a Hole, Dark Cicada, and so on.

Better yet, I thought we might as well start with Parvati's Dance. After all, I had been a Dance major. If I was going to nail any of these, this would surely be the one. I could explain it to you, but you'd probably have more fun discovering it on your own.

In typical Karin fashion, instead of being in the moment and enjoying the celebration of womanhood that Parvati represented, I fumed that there was only *one guy* pictured throughout the book— but he was with *two different* women, a blonde and a brunette. What the hell? I think it's time for an all-new feminist sex manual—*Queen Bee Sutra*. For now, all hopes of achieving orgasm had danced off and disappeared.

TWENTY-SIX

Top Seed

AFTER NINE YEARS OF DATING, JUST WHEN I THOUGHT I'D BE THE "cake" Damien got to have and eat, we became engaged. Only a year later, we were officially newlyweds. Something within me clicked. I felt a deeper connection to him than ever before. I realize this doesn't happen for everyone. Some people feel that attachment from day one, whereas others spend a lifetime searching for it. It wasn't necessarily a magical feeling, but rather, a combination of things: compatibility, closeness, and comfort with each other sexually. He had chosen to accept me for who I was—as well as who I wasn't—for the rest of our lives. This felt incredibly intimate and sexy to me.

One might think that, based on my previously detailed exploits, I had a drawerful of sexy lingerie to keep things spicy in the bedroom. This couldn't be further from the case. I didn't own much lingerie at the time and, when I did wear it, I usually turned out the lights before Damien could see me wearing it, preferring to make love in the dark.

After we got hitched, I had a total change of heart and made some hefty investments in provocative attire. Who doesn't love a little retail therapy? French maid's outfit: *check!* Stockings and garter belts: *check!* Crotchless everything: *check!* Victoria's Secret hot Mrs. Claus red hat, skirt, and bra: *check!*

I wasn't prepared for what happened next—at least, not so soon after being married.

My internal clock began beating like a drummer on steroids. My body was telling me loud and clear that I needed to pop out a bambino—pronto.

Damien liked the idea of having kids but at first wasn't sure we were ready. (Is anyone really *ready*?) After just a smidge of womanly prodding, he reluctantly agreed that we should start trying.

I went off birth control cold turkey. I held my breath, anticipating the worst. I'd heard horror stories from some of my friends who went off the pill. Mood swings galore. Massive cramps and faces turning into pepperoni pizzas. I forewarned Damien about these potential side effects, and he braced himself for a shitstorm. Luckily, I got away with only a few blemishes, although the cramps were debilitating. V had gone years without needing anything more than a junior-size tampon and suddenly I was wedging supers in to plug the flow. But, hey, it was all worth it, right?

Lo and behold, we found plenty of time for baby-making. In the morning before work. In the shower. While preparing dinner. At night after I finished work. At night after *he* finished work. In the middle of the night when his boner popped up, having decided that *it* wanted to work. To this day, I'm not sure Damien was trying to get me pregnant as much as he was just enjoying the extra excuses for sex.

The only thing getting in the way? Peanut, our puggle. He was truly the ultimate cock-blocker! Don't believe me? Let's count the ways. While Damien and I would kiss on the couch, Peanut would want to be part of the trio and lick our faces. When Damien and I would have sex in the shower, Peanut would push the bathroom door open, put his paws up on the tub, and peek in through the curtains. When Damien and I would have sex in the bedroom, the dog would scratch and claw at the door until one of us opened it. When we would try to do it on our office chair while Peanut was sleeping, he would wake up, hover in the doorway, and stare creepily at us.

I must admit, I spoiled our dog rotten. I gave him presents and cake on his birthday. I poured dog beer for him so he could drink with us. I covered him with special booties and a coat for his walks on cold days. When we visited my parents, I used a baby monitor so I could listen for him as he slept alone in a different part of the house.

I was unaware of Damien's jealousy of my relationship with the dog until one winter evening. I was dressed in cotton booty shorts and a tank top because the apartment had old radiators for heat that made the place feel like the tropics year-round. I snuggled on the couch with Peanut, kissing his nose and rubbing his belly as we watched *Meerkat Manor* on TV. (Animal Planet was Peanut's favorite station.)

Damien, who entered the room with a Corona in his hand, spoiled the Hallmark moment. His nasty eyeroll did not escape my notice (or Peanut's).

"What?" I demanded.

"Can you put the dog on the floor so I can sit with you?"

How dare he address my beloved canine in such a manner!

"The dog has a *name*—and no, I can't. As you can see, we're *snuggling*."

"You'd think you love that dog more than me," he moped.

"You're crazy. I do not," I said with a dismissive wave. I patted the couch on my left. "Look, there is plenty of room on the couch for all *three* of us."

"I don't want dog fur all over me. Just put him on the floor," he ordered.

I looked down at Peanut, who responded with a sad face. Neither of us was ready to end the snuggle. Damien and I were at an impasse. I couldn't understand why he was making such a big deal about this.

"Are you in a bad mood? Did I do something?"

"No, I'm *fine*," he said in a manner that did not sound like he was in any way fine. Suddenly, he barked, "But you spend more time with the dog and at your acting classes than you do with me!"

At last—the truth comes out. He's jealous of our dog—and my acting, too.

I didn't know how to react. I thought he adored our dog child. I thought he was supportive of my acting. Wounded and upset, I buried my face in the dog's fur.

His voice softened as he recognized that he'd gone too far. "I'm sorry I said that, I didn't mean it. Look, I love you. I love that you love acting and I love that you love Peanut. You're a really good mom to Peanut—and will be to our future child. But I need attention, too."

Wait a minute…he's right!

The realization caused me to feel wracked with guilt. I had been completely blind to how he felt. When we weren't having sex, all I did was work, attend acting classes, and play with our dog. He was looking for more of an emotional connection with me, his wife. We were still relative newlyweds, so the last thing I wanted to do was start off on the wrong foot.

Although it pained me to do so, I gently lowered Peanut to the floor. I motioned for Damien to cozy up next to me. I soothed his ego with a kiss as soon as his body landed. He tasted like beer which, inexplicably, was a total turn-on. His tongue was soft; his grip on my back was firm.

Next thing I knew, the booty shorts were calling to him and he was sweeping me off the couch and into our bedroom. Along the way, he opened the dog gate at our door with one hand while holding me up with the other. I was extra smitten at the sight of his veiny forearms.

We went into full-throttle baby-making mode. After climaxing, Damien remained inside me for a prolonged period of time to give every single sperm a fighting chance. During this interlocked lull, we started to discuss important things, such as what we were going to have for dinner or our weekend plans. About ten minutes later, he withdrew and, while still naked, went to fetch some paper towels for the cleanup. He didn't realize that the dog gate hadn't latched all of the way so, while were engrossed in our passion, Peanut had grabbed a front row seat to catch the action. After only one step, Damien tripped over Peanut; he crashed into the gate and stubbed his toe.

"This dog is going to kill me!" Damien howled.

"Well, if you sowed your seed, then I guess you're like the Brazilian slender opossum!" (They are one of the few species that die right after mating.)

I know, it was wrong of me to laugh while he was in pain—but I couldn't help myself. I did so while continuing to lie on the bed with a pillow under my butt and my legs straight up in the air. All of the books and magazine articles recommended this as the best way to help the swimmers glide downstream to reach the golden egg.

After months of nonstop action in the bedroom and elsewhere, it worked! I tested positive on a pregnancy test. To this day, both Damien and I are certain the night he stubbed his toe was when conception occurred.

This is it. I'm going to be a mom. He really does have super sperm, after all!

TWENTY-SEVEN

V Goes Dark

I suppose it was inevitable: I sold out and joined Corporate America as a sales trainer. This required a great deal of travel and meant my waving buh-bye to my acting career. (On the positive side, my days of waitressing were in the rearview mirror as well.) I ventured all over the East Coast: from Maryland to New York; from Virginia to New Jersey.

Being at the company less than a year meant I had virtually zero vacation time. At first, this didn't bother me that much. I've always been a go-getter and hyper-committed to my career—almost to the point where it nearly became a character flaw. Well…okay, it was *definitely* a character flaw. I often neglected the most important things in my life in exchange for climbing the corporate ladder. The care of my unborn baby was no exception.

In retrospect, I'm sure if I had called my boss and said, "I need to go to the doctor. The only time they can fit me in is when I'm supposed to travel to Baltimore," he would have accommodated me and shifted things around. For whatever reason—my age, inexperience, or insecurity—I just didn't feel comfortable broaching the subject. It didn't help appearances that we had a death in my family my first week on the job, causing me to exit the middle of a training session to fly home.

In this instance, I pushed an OB-GYN appointment a month out in order to accommodate attending a "Train-the-Trainer" session in Rochester, New York. (A Triple-T session was when a senior trainer did a workshop for newbies on how to deliver a new module.) I was excited about the trip because my parents were living in Rochester at the time and several of my friends from college still lived there. At the same time, I was terrified. Seemingly out of nowhere, I developed an intense anxiety about flying—probably because a living being was gestating in my belly. If something was happening to me, it was impacting our baby, too.

The day arrived for my trip to Rochester. I kissed Damien goodbye and hopped in a cab to LaGuardia Airport. It was time for work, which meant I had my game face on for the next few days.

[Dear Reader: Use your imagination to insert important business meeting activities here.]

Fast forward to two days later. I felt like garbage. I returned home to our apartment from my usual Saturday morning beauty appointments and collapsed on my bed. During my business trip, I had experienced debilitating cramps, accompanied by some blood, but shrugged it off as one last period. I think I'd read about that once in a magazine or saw it on *Oprah*. I chalked it up to my usual shitty luck.

I had been way too tied up on my business trip to find a doctor and get the issue checked out. Damien and I had agreed not to tell my parents about the pregnancy until three months in, so I wasn't about to share anything with them. In fact, I didn't tell anyone about the episode.

I curled into a tight fetal position and clenched my stomach.

Goddam, won't these cramps ever just leave me alone?

But then…

Uh-oh, emergency!

I flew into the bathroom, just a blur to Damien.

"Hey, what the—" he reacted. "Are you going to crap your pants?"

Considering I had suffered from IBS, this was a very real possibility. My pants and underwear were barely down before I saw the pooling blood. The pain in my nether regions was unbearable. I blocked out much of what happened after that, except for seeing the form of what I thought was a tiny baby on the tissue I used to wipe myself.

No, no, no! My baby! What else could it be?!

I determined that it was indeed a fetus. A motionless shell of something that should have been alive and growing inside my body.

Oh God, what do I do?

I sat on the toilet as tears poured down my face. My anguish was so unendurable that no sound accompanied my cries.

And yet, something must have triggered Damien to recognize something was wrong and knock on the door.

"Babe?" he asked in a gentle voice he saved only for potentially raw moments like this. "You okay? What's going on?"

Not knowing what else to do, I dropped the tissue in the bowl, pulled up my underwear and pants, and scrambled to open the door.

Our eyes locked. We read each other's expressions of despair and just stood there, speechless, for several seconds.

I then blurted the obvious: "I think I had a miscarriage."

He clutched me to his chest so tight I couldn't breathe. Now we both audibly cried.

Something odd happens to me when I'm around someone who is upset. I don't know why, but I feel the need to be the strong one—especially when that person is a man. At that moment, this translated into an impulsive act that continues to haunt me to this day. In order to avoid exposing Damien to the visual of what happened, I rushed over to the toilet and flicked the handle. Just like that, the remains of our offspring were gone forever. I flushed my baby.

I continue to relive that moment over and over in my mind. I can't think of much else I've done in my life that I regret more than that action. Sometimes the thought of what I did overwhelms me to the brink of being unable to function.

I returned to Damien, who was stunned by what he had just seen. "Did you just...was that—"

"It'll be okay," I assured him. "It'll be okay…."

"You have to call the doctor immediately, Karin."

Luckily, my doctor was on call that weekend. She listened as I described the situation and answered her questions.

"Are you still in pain?" the doctor asked.

"Yes, *a lot*," I replied.

"The same as while the incident occurred?"

"Yes—maybe more…."

"Get to the hospital ER *right away*. Hang up and go!" she ordered.

I did as she instructed. Damien and I became a flurry of activity, grabbing essentials, throwing Peanut some kibble, and spinning to the car. We drove from Queens to NYU Hospital in Manhattan.

We entered the ER and proceeded to the check-in window. We both became tongue-tied, not knowing what to say. The nurse looked up from her desk, handed me a form on a clipboard with a pen, and brayed, "What are you here for?"

Again, the words didn't come out.

Oh, ya know, I just lost my baby and then freaked out and flushed it down the toilet. Thought I should get checked out, since it feels like one hundred knives cutting my insides to pieces. On second thought, I probably shouldn't say that….

I cleared my throat and whispered, "Um, I think I had a miscarriage. My doctor told me to come in right away. I'm having really bad cramps, and they won't go away."

"Oh, I'm sorry," she empathized. "Did you bring the fetus?"

Fetus? Was I supposed to? Why would I have thought to do that? What would I have put it—or should I say "him" or "her"—in? A baggie?

"No," I answered, my hands trembling with the clipboard.

"Okay—have a seat, and we'll call you shortly."

I nodded my head, retreating to an available seat with the clipboard. Once again, I fought back the tears. Part of me mourned my baby; part of me dealt with the excruciating pain; and a third part was wracked with guilt for having pressed that toilet bowl lever.

No matter what your situation might be entering an ER, the wait always seems longer than it should be. What if I were dying or something? There was nothing Damien and I could say to each other that would make this situation any better, so, after completing the form, I clutched his hand and stared at the wall.

An hour later, a nurse finally called me into a room where she checked my vitals and questioned me about what had happened. This particular nurse was kind and supportive, so I felt a bit less tense. On top of that, my preliminary readings were all normal. Since the ER was backed up and all beds filled, I returned to the waiting room and opted for magazine page-flipping.

Wouldn't you know it—an article about the best ways to get pregnant. Thanks.

Another half hour went by until a bed was ready. The nurse screeched the curtain around me so I would have privacy as I stripped down and pulled on the ratty hospital gown. Try as I might, I could not tie the back strings, which meant my back and butt were exposed.

Ugh, I wish I had a private room right about now.

I felt like a child as Damien dutifully tied the strings into bows. I lay down on the bed but couldn't get comfortable. The pain was continuing to mount. Once again, Damien came to the rescue and rubbed my back.

"As soon as the doctor comes in, can you ask him if I can have some pain medication?" I asked.

"Sure," Damien obliged.

The doctor said "knock knock" with an exaggerated shake of the curtain. "Come in," Damien and I invited.

"What do we have here?" the doctor mumbled to himself as he reviewed the chart. He looked like the real deal: tall, thin, well-groomed, round glasses, stethoscope, and white coat with tie underneath.

Damien took the opportunity to charge right in. "Doctor, is it possible to prescribe some medication for her right away? She's in a lot of pain."

Please, please, please…just a couple of Extra Strength Advil will do.

"I have to examine her first and run a few tests," the doctor answered. "We'll probably need to conduct a vaginal ultrasound to see what's going on."

Come on, can't you see I'm dying here?!

The doctor completed his examination, during which—yet again—I had to explain that I had flushed what might have been my child down the toilet. He was professional and nonjudgmental throughout the exchange. After scribbling something on the chart, he rolled up a chair next to me and sat. He didn't seem to mind that his back leaned far into the curtain—probably bugging the patient next door. His hand went on my wrist. "I'm sorry you've had such a traumatic experience," he said in a low tone. "We definitely need to do the ultrasound."

"What is it? What happened?" Damien and I asked.

"I can't say for sure yet, but I believe you have had an ectopic pregnancy. This occurs when the egg is fertilized in the fallopian tube instead of in the uterus. The baby eventually runs out of room and can't grow any further."

Both Damien and I brought our hands to our mouths in shock. Even though we knew it was unlikely going to be good news, it still felt a lot more official and graver coming from the doctor. "If it is an ectopic pregnancy, there can be *very serious* risks to the mother—so we have to handle this delicately. This is why you can't have any medication. We'll monitor your pain level while we wait for the vaginal ultrasound to be ready."

Very serious risks? Does he mean what I think he means?

If I was panicking before, now I was really over the edge. During the wait for the ultrasound, my pain level worsened by about ten times. An hour or so later, I was led through the cold hospital hallway to a private room for the test.

I can assure you this is fact: Nothing is more humiliating than having a male doctor give you a vaginal ultrasound. First, he takes out a gigantic wand that essentially resembles a penis. He unrolls a rubber cover—aka a wand condom—over it. He lubes up the shaft with some KY Jelly. Now it's fun time! The wand penetrates the vagina, shifts around, and rotates in a variety of angles to get pictures.

"*Hey, watch where you're going under the hood with that thing, buddy!*" V burst out.

I struck back: "*Oh, so now you speak up! Where were you when I needed a little heads-up that something was wrong?*"

"*Look, we've never been pregnant before. How was I supposed to know?*"

She had a point. I allowed her to have the last word and returned to sulking.

When all was said and done, the doctor confirmed that I did indeed have an ectopic pregnancy. However, he couldn't verify that everything was out of me. He and the nurses barraged me with questions about what I had seen on the tissue, but I started second-guessing myself. I had been so discombobulated I didn't know for sure whether it was a partial or complete fetus.

Everyone continued to emphasize that this was an extremely dangerous situation. I had to remain in the hospital overnight to be monitored. If the pain were to continue or if I were to have more bleeding, they might need to perform laparoscopic surgery to remove any additional parts of the fetus.

The doctor stepped out to secure a room for me—and not a moment too soon. I broke down as soon the door closed. The doctors had referred to my baby as if it were never a living, breathing human being.

How can they be so insensitive?

By this time, it was after 11:00 PM. I just wanted to be home in my own bed, holding Peanut and snuggling with Damien. A private NYU hospital room would have to do. Damien curled up in a chair in the corner of our room, leaving me alone in bed with dark thoughts for who knows how long.

Just twenty-four hours ago I was pregnant—a mom-to-be. Where did it all go wrong? Why did this have to happen to me? Why didn't I go to the doctor sooner?

Would our baby have been a boy or a girl? Who would the child have looked more like—Damien or me? What would we have named him or her? Now that I think about it…maybe we should name the baby anyway? My God, we can't even have a proper burial.

I lost track of time but, at some point, my eyelids became so heavy they could no longer resist closing for the evening. The next thing I knew, a new nurse was waking me up to check my vitals and run a pregnancy test, the single most important requirement before I could leave. The results came back negative.

I didn't know how to process this news except I felt some measure of relief that at least I was out of the woods and could be released. I looked toward the corner, where Damien was motionless in the chair. I figured he was exhausted and gave him every ounce of well-deserved sleep before we could leave.

Meanwhile, I removed the gown in one swift motion, discarding it as if it were trash. I finished dressing just as the nurse handed me the discharge papers.

After I finished reviewing and signing the paperwork, it was time to go—except Damien was *still* down for the count. I half-heartedly chuckled to myself in admiration of his ability to sleep anywhere amidst anything and gently woke him up.

Dazed and emotionally drained, we exited the hospital into the glaring daylight toward our parked car. We drove up to the cashier window to pay when we were greeted by another unpleasant surprise.

"Forty-eight fifty," the cashier said, reviewing our ticket.

Fifty bucks?! You've got to be fucking kidding me!

PART 6

No Vacancy

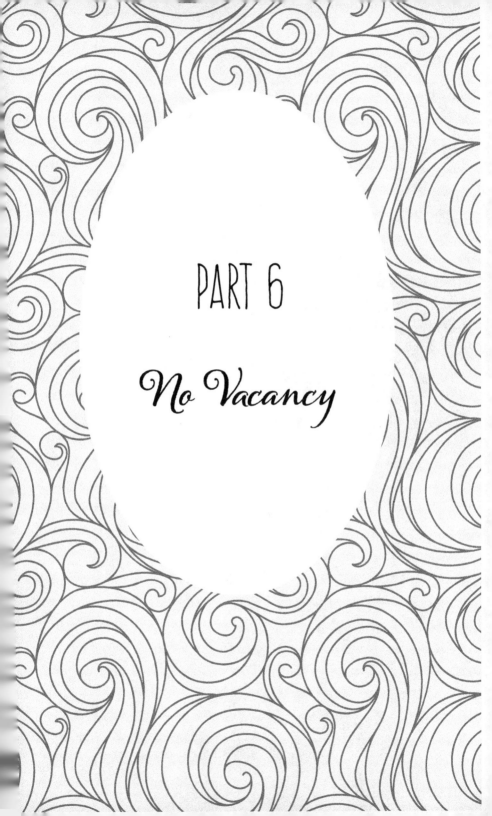

*W*ho knew I'd find solace in a quote from Eeyore: "Could be worse. Not sure how, but it could be." He was right and each day it got a little easier.

Damien and I were hands-off each other for several weeks but, humans being humans—and V being V—eventually we all developed the itch to get back to business. One day, our sex drives returned with a vengeance and all I could think about was getting pregnant again. My quest for the Big O would have to shift to the back burner. Apparently, my body was unable to focus on two things at once.

This time, I vowed, when it happens, I will be more careful and not take any unnecessary risks. I'm a responsible adult, I'm a responsible adult, I'm a responsible adult. Right, V?

"Yeah, yeah, totally responsible," V reflected. "Just let me at your hubby's broomstick!"

TWENTY-EIGHT

Maybe Baby

ONE THING I WILL NEVER UNDERSTAND: HOW IS IT POSSIBLE FOR A woman to not know she is pregnant until a head is popping out of her vagina? Every once in a while, I hear or read about a story that goes something like this: "I went into the hospital to have a cyst removed and came home with twins—it's a miracle!"

I can, however, appreciate a woman's not knowing she's pregnant while still in the early days. In order for a woman to recognize this so early, she must be super-attuned to her body and have pinpoint accuracy predicting her period—things I was clearly lacking.

I happened to be in Virginia for a training session with our sales account executives for three days. Upon arrival at the training office, my colleagues and I were greeted by a sizable ant infestation. We called the building exterminator to pay us a visit and evict the creatures as soon as possible.

The exterminator—a Mr. T lookalike (for those who recall *The A-Team* TV show) but without the mohawk and far gentler in nature—arrived during my group's lunchtime. He entered lugging a gas mask and his extermination gear. He spotted us around a table attempting to eat our sandwiches while fighting a losing battle against the swarming ant army.

"Excuse me!" he addressed us. "Any of you ladies pregnant or possibly pregnant?"

No, of course not. I'm already on my second latte—how could I be pregnant?

I gave the matter a second thought before opening my mouth. The truth was: I really didn't know. Damien and I were trying, so it was *possible.* I felt totally normal, having zero telltale signs, such as morning sickness. Then again, it had been a while since I'd had my last period. I tried counting on my fingers to figure out when it was, but I got confused the moment I needed a third hand.

Meanwhile, the women around the table were nodding and uttering emphatic "No's." All eyes landed on me, accompanied by silence. The exterminator hovered over me, staring me down.

Do I look pregnant to him? Is he an expert on life as well as death?

I scrunched my face and asked, "What if…you don't know if you're pregnant or not?"

He folded his muscular arms. "Ma'am," he declared, "I can't spray this room until we know if you're pregnant."

"Um…what happens if you spray and it turns out I'm pregnant?"

"Exposure could cause bad things to happen to the fetus," he replied. "You don't want to know."

Really? Like the baby will sprout a sixth toe or grow up to be a politician?

"It looks like we have about forty-five minutes before our class starts," I considered, checking my watch. "I guess I could run to the drugstore and buy a quick pregnancy test."

"Yes ma'am, good idea," he acknowledged. "I suggest you do that. I'll come back in an hour."

The women chuckled to themselves as I locked up my laptop and grabbed my keys and purse. "Where are you going to do the test? In the gross bathroom here?" Laura, a coworker, asked.

I haven't considered that yet….

"Yeah," I answered. "I guess so."

I zoomed off to the drugstore in my rental car, gulping down the remains of what I hoped wouldn't be my last latte for months. I hurried inside, heading straight to the pregnancy test aisle. There were two shelves of options, priced between five and twenty dollars.

I struggled to make a decision. They all looked the same.

Is this a situation where the phrase "you get what you pay for" applies?

Running low on funds and pressed for time, I had to choose. This became especially difficult as I realized the cashier was squinting down at me from her perch at the register. I guessed she was in her early sixties, as she had whitened hair, a mess of wrinkles, and a few indiscernible skin marks on her face.

Uh, here goes nothing!

I impulsively grabbed the "middle of the road"-priced test, figuring it had to work better than the cheapo ones and that I didn't need the expensive designer model to show off to anyone.

I knew I was in for it as soon as I started my approach to the cashier. She'd been scrutinizing me all along, but now her furrowed eyebrows were undoubtedly scrutinizing me. Although I was dressed in corporate clothes, I was tiny and could still pass to some people as a teenager.

"Mn-hmn," she judged, eyeing my purchase on the counter.

I knew I should have gotten a few other things to distract her from the pregnancy test. Maybe it's not too late to get a pack of Bubble Yum?

"Got yourself into some trouble, eh dear?"

"Trouble? What do you mean?"

"I see it all the time—you young girls coming in here for these tests."

"I'm old, well...not as old as you," I spouted. "Wait, that didn't come out right."

I searched into my purse for my wallet, needing something to focus my attention on—anything other than her. "I just turned twenty-eight, in fact. I'm trying to get pregnant. I even have ID somewhere in here as proof."

"You ought to learn to respect your elders," she reprimanded me.

"I'm sorry, I'm in a hurry...."

She rolled her eyes before scanning the pregnancy test box.

"Aren't they always. Twelve seventy-five is your total."

Fortunately, I had exact change and didn't have to wait for her to fumble in the register. As I turned away, she asked: "You want a bag?"

"No thanks," I replied, continuing toward the automatic doors and cramming my purchase into my purse.

"What about a receipt? Don't you want your receipt? You'll need it if you have to return it."

Return it? Who returns a used pregnancy test?

"I'm good, thank you!" I exclaimed, shooting out before she had a chance to ask yet another irritating question.

Upon returning to the office, I headed straight for the bathroom. Thankfully, all of the stalls were empty and the sliding lock worked without any issue. I ripped open the packaging of the pregnancy test and scanned the directions.

Pee on stick—got it. Wait three minutes—gross, but fine. Look at stick. If the + sign comes up, I'm pregnant. If the − sign comes up, I'm not. Whatever happened to "blue" means "pregnant"? Whatever—seems easy enough.

I dropped my pants and panties before beginning my descent into a squat. I hovered for a moment, using my left arm to prop myself up on the toilet paper roll; meanwhile, my right hand had to do the dirty work of positioning the stick under the stream. Except for one problem—V cracked under the pressure.

"Oh, come on, just pee already!" I howled at her.

"Hey, lay off," V countered. "*I can't function under such conditions.*"

"Seriously? *There's no one here but us. Would you like me to run some water for you, Your Highness?*"

"Yeah, actually, that might do the trick!"

I groaned while pulling my underwear back up. I unbolted the door and slid toward the sink while still clutching the stick.

"*You really are a diva, ya know that?*"

"*Do you want me to pee or not?*"

I turned both faucets on to produce a steady flow and returned to the stall. I repeated all of my prior preparations and waited...and waited. As seconds ticked by, my thigh muscles weakened and my legs teetered.

"V, I don't know how much longer I can hold this position...."

"I need more motivation."

"More motivation?!"

"Yeah," she said. "How about thinking some wet thoughts—like the time we broke the sink boinking that hot college dude. We caused some flood!"

"We sure did, but I'm married now. I can't be thinking about that! How about the time we went to Niagara Falls in elementary school? Make like the Maid of the Mist already!"

"It's a lot less sexy—but I'll try."

V let loose a geyser. My pee gushed all over the stick, my hand, the seat—and my pants.

"For fuck's sake, V!"

"Sorry, I guess I got carried away. Maybe if you'd laid off the lattes this wouldn't be happening!"

The monsoon beneath me continued, unabated; once V got started, it was nearly impossible for her to stop. My legs were about to buckle, so I just gave up and sat on the toilet while ensuring I didn't drop the stick in the bowl or cause any more spillage on myself. At last, the final droplets splashed down and I could start the timer.

Three minutes, right? You'd think technology could determine this a lot faster these days.

I knew that the two worst things for me to do were 1) look at the stick as it performed its magic; or 2) stare at my watch, as it would make the passing time seem even longer.

My mind drifted...

What if I find out I'm pregnant now? How will I tell Damien? Should I call him right away? He'll want to know, for sure. Or...maybe I should *just wait until I get home so I can see the reaction on his face, and we can share the moment together.*

I regained focus just as my watch reached the final countdown: *four, three, two...one!*

Ready or not, here I come!

I looked at it with one slanted eye: *negative.*

Really?

I looked at it with both eyes wide open.

Yep, negative.

I was relieved and saddened at the same time. On the one hand, I had been looking forward to finding out I had a party for one in my belly. On the other, it wasn't much of a surprise. Nothing about my body felt remotely pregnant. I tossed the pregnancy test in the tampon receptacle before zipping up, stepping out, and washing my hands—with lots and lots of liquid soap.

Did I just take a pregnancy test at work? Yep—classy!

I reemerged in the classroom. My colleagues stopped in their tracks to read my facial expression and body language.

"So...are you knocked up?"

"Nope, not yet," I said through a fake smile. "Let's blast those little terrors!"

Everyone cheered and applauded. When Mr T. returned to commence spraying, we vacated the area. Several minutes later, we returned to the odor-filled room; the spray remained in the air for the rest of the day. On the positive side, the ants were toast.

A couple of weeks later, I found out that I had indeed been pregnant that afternoon. Either the test had been contaminated and/or faulty, or I had a false negative result because it was too early to make a determination.

Fucking "middle of the road" test!

Then I had a genuine concern: I'd had exposure to that bug-killing spray for at least four hours. What if my child were to be born with six toes, after all?

TWENTY-NINE

Womb There It Is

YOU WOULD THINK THAT, AFTER THOUSANDS OF YEARS OF WOMEN trying to determine if they are pregnant and all of the innovation we've witnessed over the past three decades, someone would have come up with a better method to confirm a pregnancy than peeing on a stick. How disgusting is it to place a urine-soaked test strip on the bathroom counter and then wait three minutes for the result? I mean, I brush my teeth and do my makeup there!

I may have been a bit premature in revealing how I found out that I was pregnant. Allow me to backtrack and lay out how the night went down.

It'd been a long week for both of us at our respective jobs. I had been traveling for three weeks straight—one each in Virginia, Maryland, and Pennsylvania. I barely had time to settle into our new home in New Jersey. I was used to living out of suitcases—but doing so out of boxes was driving me crazy.

On Friday night, Damien and I crashed on the couch in front of the TV with a fine bottle of pinot noir. (By "fine," I mean that it was drinkable and under twelve dollars.) I broke out a box of carefully packaged stemware, from which I selected two appropriate glasses. Damien uncorked the bottle and filled my glass all the way up to the top.

I took a nice big swig of the wine, allowing the taste to linger in my mouth for a moment before swallowing it down. I smacked my lips. It was beyond delicious.

I deserve this glass of wine. But...wait. Maybe I should take a quick pregnancy test before drinking more? Nah, how bad could one drink be? Besides, red wine is good for your heart, right?

I took another sip.

But...I already had one miscarriage. Do I really want to risk another?

I placed my glass on the coffee table and turned to Damien. "Do you think I should take a pregnancy test?"

He perked right up. "Why—do you think you're pregnant?"

"I don't know. I haven't had my period in a while...since before Virginia."

"Well...are you late?"

"I don't know," I shrugged.

"What do you mean you don't know? How do you not know if you're late?"

"Cuz—I don't track it, and it never comes on time anyway. My cycle isn't normal."

He reacted in befuddlement at my utter lack of understanding about how my body worked.

"I took a test when I was in Virginia about three weeks ago. Definitely seems like I should have had my period by now."

"Well, I guess you better check—just to be safe."

I ventured into the bathroom, wine glass in hand, to find a pregnancy test from under the bathroom sink. I had been buying so many of the middle-to-high price range tests from the drugstore the past ten months that the expense was driving us broke. Given that I'd already peed on and disposed of so many sticks with only negative results to show for my efforts, I now opted for the cheapos from the Dollar Store. By that point, a buck seemed like just the right price for a useless pee stick. Too bad you can't put it in the recycling bin. There must be loads of those things piling up in landfills.

I went through my usual routine: pants down; butt plop on the seat; tear open the test; maneuver stick under the stream to avoid splashes; place test on top of tissues on the sink; blah-blah-blah.

As usual, I attempted to avoid peeking before time was up but couldn't resist. My eyes locked on the test as I zipped up my jeans.

Whoa! What's this? A line and then another line?

This is really it! We're pregnant! We did it, V!

I held back a joyful scream because I wanted to surprise Damien. I frantically practiced selecting the perfect words and making the right facial expression while looking at myself in the mirror.

Babe, it's positive!

We're having a baby!

I hope you like me thick because I'm about to blow up!

Your wand worked its magic!

Your baby batter is in the oven!

Although none of these announcements seemed right, I couldn't keep the news to myself any longer. When I swung open the bathroom door, I was surprised to find him standing and waiting for me.

"So, what's it say?"

All of my rehearsed facial expressions went out the window, replaced by a doofus grin. I shoved the glistening wet stick in front of his nose.

"Get that thing away from me," he remarked, stepping back a few inches while eyeing the result. By this time, he had become educated enough to distinguish a positive from negative. His face lit up with excitement as he wrapped himself around me. I enjoyed the tight squeeze until my eyeballs felt like they were going to pop out of my head.

We jumped up and down like giddy children when I spotted my wine glass and had several traumatic realizations.

Oh no—what have I done? I might have been pregnant when the exterminator sprayed the room! I got high from the fumes when we painted the house last weekend! I just drank wine! This baby is already doomed to have six toes, antennae, and a hump!

As you've probably gathered by now, I wasn't one to always follow my inner voice and do what was practical and safe. The opposite irresistible impulse took over, drawing me to my glass of wine.

My hand reached over to take one final celebratory swig.

What the hell, one more sip won't make any difference now.

A hand snatched the glass away from lips just in the nick of time. "I'll be finishing that," Damien volunteered.

And, just like that, I waved *sayonara* to my drinking days. Luckily, I had quit smoking a few years earlier or I would have been going through major withdrawal. From here on out, I was relegated to prenatal vitamins, Smartwater…and the occasional O'Doul's nonalcoholic beer.

THIRTY

All Lubed Up with Nowhere to Go

WHAT'S NOT TO LOVE ABOUT BEING PREGNANT?

This was my main thought during the first few months while V was making her glorious transition to becoming a womb. My breasts were gigantic—a full 34C, if not a D. I ate whatever crazy food I wanted—not weird things like ice cream with pickles or bacon with mustard or pizza with chocolate sauce—but Ritz crackers and ruby red grapefruit juice. I devoured sleeves of Ritz until my taste buds turned numb from the salt.

Around seven months into the pregnancy, I waddled into my OB-GYN's office for a routine checkup, expecting it to be like any other visit: check my weight; take my blood pressure; remind me to eat healthy foods; and maybe get an idea of when the gross mucus plug I'd heard about was going to make its grand appearance. Then I'd hobble back to my car and be on my way.

Not so! Dr. Decker had other plans in store for me.

I arrived on time and spent the requisite twenty minutes in the waiting room glumly staring at pictures of super fit celebrity bodies in women's magazines. I had been so excited to start showing but, once I did, I longed to have my old body back. It seemed like my belly was never going to stop expanding. Most of all, I missed looking at V. I could barely see over my belly to weed her garden. I hoped the overgrown bush wouldn't suffocate her.

A nurse called out my name. I set the magazine down and shuffled into an examination room. "Have a seat on the table," she directed. "Everything off from the waist down. Here's a cover for your lap."

She handed me a thin paper blanket to help conceal my nether regions and exited the room.

I began to disrobe my lower half....

Damn—I knew I should have tried to shave down there this morning.

I shed the rest of my clothes and used all of my energy to hoist myself up on the table. Once I finally made it, I struggled to catch my breath.

Dr. Decker entered not a moment too soon; the paper underneath my butt was already starting to stick to my skin.

"Hi, Karin. How are you feeling today?" she asked in a bubbly voice.

"Ya know, like I smoked a pack of cigarettes and just ran a marathon."

She laughed and instructed me to lie on my back. As I did so she added, "Let's check your cervix and see how things are looking."

"Great, I hope you know where the cervix is, because I don't," I remarked, allowing my head to fall back against the pillow. I raised my legs into the stirrups while scooting down towards the edge of the table.

I'm all saddled up—yeehaw!

She went about her normal business examining my cervix and other miscellaneous things until her head popped out from my abyss. "Everything looks good. You're not dilating yet, which is good. Now, we should talk about preparing your body for the birth."

"Oh yeah, I'm taking a Lamaze class," I proudly stated.

"That's good—but it's not what I meant. You need to start stretching your skin out so you don't tear."

"Tear?"

"Yes," she nodded. "Some women tear when they give birth if the baby's head is larger than the skin can stretch to accommodate it. Don't worry, I'll show you what to do. It's quite simple."

She began her demonstration as she spoke, mimicking pouring olive oil on her hand. "You want to take some olive oil and place it on your two fingers."

Ugh. Where is she going with this?

"Then you're going to lather it on the skin at the opening of your vagina by making a half-circle motion on the lower side. Like so."

Her fingers swung side-to-side like a pendulum.

This sounds gross. Maybe V wants a salad down there?

"Got it?" she asked.

"Yeah, sure, got it."

There's no way I'm ever doing this. Thanks for the advice, doc lady, but you're crazy!

The visit concluded and I got dressed. On my way to the car, I couldn't help think my doctor had lost her mind. Did she really believe I was going to start massaging olive oil all over my lady parts?

Not a chance.

☾ ☉ ☾

Damien had started working the second shift to make extra money, so on most days we were like passing ships. Since it was a Friday night, I decided to wait up for him to arrive, which would be around midnight. I found a comfy spot on the couch and nuzzled up to Peanut as best as I could with my ever-expanding belly, a sleeve of Ritz crackers in one hand and the remote in the other. I channel surfed for a while and couldn't land on anything of interest. Boredom set in right away, which enabled V to raid my thoughts.

"*Hey—remember that olive oil thing? It sounds kind of interesting. I was thinking maybe we could give that a shot.*"

"What? Really? Why?"

"*Well, for starters, I'm not too excited about tearing. But I also think* the olive oil might feel nice. It'll really soften up the skin—maybe bring back some of my youthful glow."

"You're still youthful, V—aren't you?"

"The fact that you asked that means you haven't been paying me enough attention lately," she criticized.

"Sorry, V. Been kinda busy with work and building a baby."

"I know, but I've been getting stir-crazy down here. What do you have to lose trying out something new?"

"Nothing, I guess…."

"Great, lube me up!"

I hoisted myself off the couch and headed for the kitchen. I pulled the oils out of the cabinet and lined them up on the counter. "Let's see what we've got," I muttered to myself. "Olive oil…canola oil… grapeseed oil. I wonder if it really matters which one. I'm not sure I want to use the good stuff—olive oil is expensive."

"Bring on the extra virgin stuff!"

"What a joke, V—you're anything but a virgin. But, since you've been feeling neglected, I suppose I can splurge this once. Don't say I never do anything for you."

We kept the extra virgin olive oil—which we generally used for salads and to drizzle on bread—in a small glass container that had a nozzle at the top. Seemed like this would be easier to use that than the original large bottle. Off I went to the bathroom with the container in hand.

Now what? I know—I need a towel. This might get messy.

I grabbed a bath towel from a hook and spread it out on the edge of the bathtub. Not only would it catch any drips, it would be softer on my backside. I removed my maternity pants.

I was about to sit and get down to business when V interjected, "Maybe we should set the mood."

"Set the mood!" I fired back.

"Yeah—lights out. Maybe a candle."

"A candle! This isn't a date. It's supposed to be preventive medicine— you know, doctor recommended."

"*Sure it is,*" V mocked. "*If that's true, why do I feel like we're already starting to get off on the idea?*"

She had a point. "*All right, V, I suppose a little aroma would be nice.*"

I rummaged around the house for a candle, but all I could find was a Christmas cookie-scented one. It would have to do. I turned off the light, lit the candle, and inhaled some holiday cheer.

"*Nice,*" V cooed. "*Now let's start spreading some oil!*"

I disrobed down to my bra and carefully positioned myself on the towel. I set the olive oil container on the toilet lid.

"*I'm going to have to disinfect this container when we're done.*"

"*Less chitchat, more action. Moisten up those fingers and do that pendulum thing the doc showed us.*"

V was getting impatient, which meant I had little time to waste. I tipped the olive oil container against my fingers. In my eagerness, I must have tilted the angle too far; before I knew what was happening, olive oil was dripping all over my toes.

Oh no, that came out way too fast! What do I do with all this extra?

I slapped my coated fingers against V's exterior. I couldn't afford to waste another drop, which was expensive and creating a mess.

V began to throw a tantrum: "*That isn't the pendulum! I want the pendulum!*"

"*I know, I know—hold on...it's not as easy as it looked!*"

I tried my best to get my hands to face inward, like the doctor had shown me. I lifted my left leg and placed it on the toilet lid. I contorted my hands to simulate the pendulum motion.

My greasy foot slipped, knocking the olive oil container on the tile. A generous portion of liquid splashed across the floor. Fortunately, the glass didn't break. As I leaned forward to pick up the container, the towel slid off the edge of the tub, taking me with it.

My knees thudded against the tile floor.

"Ouch!"

"*Why are you on all fours? That's not how the doctor did it,*" V remarked.

"No shit, V. I could use a little help here. My arms aren't long enough to get my fingers in the right position. Maybe if I put the olive oil on the backside of my fingers and try to rub it on that way?"

"Yeah, let's try that. Get back up on the towel!"

I repositioned myself on the towel for a second attempt. Although I'd wasted a good portion of olive oil, I didn't feel the necessary amount was on my fingers and, being more careful this time, trickled a few drops on them. I gave the pendulum motion a go.

"Huh," V considered. "This isn't exactly what I had in mind. Are you supposed to be stretching me this far?"

"I don't know—but an eight-or-so-pound baby is going to come shooting out of you, so yeah, I probably need to stretch you this far. For the record, I'm not enjoying this, either."

"You need to file your nails, woman! You're scratching me. Forget about enjoyment—this just plain sucks!"

I tried for a few more seconds, but it just didn't feel like I was doing it right. V and I weren't getting any pleasure out of this and I seriously doubted I was making enough progress, despite the discomfort. I couldn't imagine V was getting any more supple and youthful looking than when we started. I began to get frustrated, tired, and out of breath. All I could think about was all the messes I had made—on the floor, on the towel, and all over myself—and whether the doctor had pranked me.

"Let's bag it, V," I said. "Let's just have positive thoughts that there won't be any tearing. Hopefully small heads run in the family...or loose vaginas!"

I wiped the excess olive oil off myself and put my clothes back on. I knew I should have showered and cleaned the floor, but I was drained. I barely had enough strength left to blow out the candle. Before long, I was back on the couch channel surfing with Peanut and wolfing down Ritz crackers. After the fifth cracker, the olive oil smell on my fingers caused me to lose my appetite, and I shoved the package aside.

Damien arrived home right on time, at midnight. "Hi," he said, kissing the top of my head. "Did you have a good night?" He was already halfway to the bathroom before I could respond.

"What the hell happened in here?!" he shouted. "Why is the olive oil in the bathroom?"

I waited for him to finish his business and come out of the bathroom before responding. Desperate for an answer to his question, he raced toward me while still zipping up his fly. "So?" he asked.

"Well," I began, trying to find the right words that would save me from seeming like I was completely clueless. "I tried to do this thing my doctor recommended, so I wouldn't tear when I have the baby. It didn't go *quite* the way it was supposed to go."

"Yeah, I can see that!"

"It was real easy for the doctor to do it because she was facing me. I can't get my fingers in my vagina the same way."

"Oh my God, you know what you need to do?" he asked with a straight face. "You should write a book and call it *I Don't Know My Vagina*—clearly, you have no idea how that thing works."

I let out a belly laugh. "That's the dumbest thing I've ever heard. Who would want to read a book about my vagina?"

"Every other woman who doesn't know how her vagina works," he answered. "Unless you're the only one out there. I mean—I don't get that you don't know how it works. I know *exactly* how my penis works."

"It's not the same—vaginas are tricky!"

"You amaze me, Karin. I hope you figure this mom thing out better than your vagina."

"Me too—or we're doomed!"

THIRTY-ONE

Ticking Time Bomb

WHEN YOU'RE PREGNANT, EVERYONE WANTS TO GIVE YOU ADVICE. Some of it will be good, some of it will be bad. Things that may sound crazy at first—like setting your baby in a car seat on the dryer (because he likes the vibration and it will soothe him to sleep)—suddenly seem brilliant when you are sleep-deprived and your infant is screaming for four hours straight in the middle of the night. I advise this: Listen to all of it, apply the things you like, and toss out the rest.

Then there are those tidbits that aren't as black-and-white and require some additional homework.

To get an episiotomy or not? That is the question. (Well, there is another question for non-Jews—*to circumcise or not to circumcise*— but we'll tackle that some other time.)

Now, just in case you don't know what an episiotomy is, let me save you a Google click. This is a procedure done when the doctor makes a nice clean slit with a surgical knife between the back of your vagina and your anus during the birthing process. *Why might a doctor do such a horrific-sounding thing,* you ask? Hold that thought: We'll get to it...eventually.

To understand my predicament, you need to go all the way back to 1980, when I was born, and the moments leading up to when I was pushed out of my mom's vagina. Doesn't that all sound so magical? Um…nope. Apparently, she gave birth to me *without any drugs*—and, yes, they were available in those days.

My mom carried on the fine tradition of natural births from my grandmother, who popped out *seven* kids naturally—some of whom were *big* babies! My mom seemed to convey a sense that there wasn't much to it, so I gave some consideration to skipping the drugs—but with wiggle room to change my mind, if things were to become unbearable.

My mom did give me one emphatic warning—one that I regret not having investigated further before following. "No matter what," she said, "*Do not* get the episiotomy!"

The horror was almost too much to bear! She recounted in graphic detail how the doctors had sliced her stretched flesh to make room for the baby's head—*my* head, that is—and how she felt every inch of the knife as it ripped its way to her anus. And that was just for starters. The worst part, according to her, was the recovery from the episiotomy. She could barely sit on a toilet for days without feeling searing pain. The image of this scared me shitless (as it were). It only took that one description for me to adamantly decline the episiotomy.

She's my mom. She had two babies without any drugs. This lady knows a thing or two about how to manage your vagina in a birthing situation… right?

Thanks to my mom's nugget of wisdom, I decided to make a birth plan. As it happened, this was a trendy thing to do at the time. I kept a copy of it for posterity, which I now bestow upon you…

••••••••••••••••••••• BIRTH PLAN •••••••••••••••••••••

Damien and I appreciate your help and expertise as we embark on this birthing experience. While we understand that last-minute situations may arise, we would like to follow this below birthing plan as closely as possible. Thank you!

LABOR

✔ I would like to labor from home as long as possible.

✔ Upon arrival to the hospital, I would like to remain as mobile as possible with intermittent monitoring, if permitted. I would like the ability to walk the halls if I need to move.

✔ I will request epidural or pain medication when needed, but prefer not to have any at all, if possible.

DELIVERY

✔ I would not like to have an episiotomy, unless medically necessary for the health and well-being of myself or the baby.

✔ Perform a C-section only if medically necessary for the health and well-being of myself or the baby.

✔ I would like to use a birthing ball and birthing bar and be as mobile as possible during labor. I would like the flexibility to choose the position I feel most comfortable in—whether it be squatting, lying on my side, etc.

✔ Only doctors and nurses are welcome in the delivery room. Absolutely no medical students, spectators, etc.

✔ I would like to keep a dim, quiet, and calm room with the door shut at all times.

POST-BIRTH

✔ The father would like to cut the umbilical cord.

✔ We would like to collect cord blood.

✔ I would like to hold and breastfeed as soon as possible after giving birth.

✔ We would like our son to room-in with me at all times.

✔ We would like to circumcise our son (with local anesthesia). Damien would like to be present for the circumcision, if possible.

• •

The most important thing to know about a birth plan is this: *Count on never actually using it.* There will be Murphy's Law at work with your birthing experience, so be prepared to improvise. This is how it went down for me....

⑥ ⑨ ⑩

Thanksgiving, 2009. My husband's entire family were invited to our house. This was a pretty exciting event for us, as it marked our first Thanksgiving in our new home. Damien looked forward to show-ing off his turkey-cooking skills, which included brining our turkey overnight and making all the fixings—mashed potatoes, yams, stuff-ing, biscuits, green beans, and cranberry sauce. The festive meal was sure to be a hit!

As for the baby: Although I was huge, I felt as if I had some time left to go because, technically, I wasn't due for another two weeks. (Forecasting date of birth is, after all, an exact science, isn't it?) My cervix had dilated a few inches, but I felt fine—assuming that "fine" meant being stabbed in the sciatic nerve every time I sat down and being unable to bend down and tie my shoelaces.

Although I could barely reach over my belly to get to the sink, I soldiered on and hand-washed every piece of china for the meal.

Deep down, I prayed that two things would not occur before carv-ing into the turkey and by the time everyone had completed dessert:

1. My water breaking.
2. The mucus plug dropping.

How hard could it be to keep those couple of things in check?

Fortunately for me, not hard at all. Our first Thanksgiving was an unbridled success. We made it through Thanksgiving without having a baby!

1. Family arguments: zilch.
2. Broken glassware or dishware: nothing.
3. Spillage: zero.
4. Water breaking: nada.
5. Mucus plug dropping: nope.

Damien and I were exhausted from all of the preparations and cleanup. My feet had swollen two sizes over the course of the day, so we decided to pack it in for the evening. I was out before my unwashed face hit the pillow.

2:34 AM: I inexplicably woke up.

Ugh, what am I doing awake right now? Well—I might as well get up and pee.

As I sat up, I felt something wet on my legs. I touched the bedding.

Oh yeah, that's wet alright. Damn it—I've peed the bed! I really should have invested in some Depends.

I sat on the edge of the bed to ponder the situation for a moment.

Do I wake Damien and tell him I peed the bed? That's kind of gross. Can't imagine him being thrilled with this news in the middle of his rest. Maybe I'll leave it for the morning and sleep somewhere else—after I shower.

I summoned up enough energy to lift myself off the bed and head to the bathroom. I sat on the toilet and peed...and peed...and peed...

Hmn. How can I have this much pee when I just peed the bed?

I leaned my head toward my pajama pants and underwear to smell my pajama bottom. *Hmn. That doesn't smell like pee—does it? Wait! Maybe...*

I took another whiff to confirm my suspicion.

…my water broke?

I had no idea what "broken water" smells like, but I knew pretty well that the liquid covering me was not just any ordinary pee.

Yes, that's it! My water broke! Thank God—I didn't pee the bed! I'm redeemed!

Oh my gosh, I wonder if this baby is going to come soon.

I flushed the toilet and washed my hands. I yawned and stretched while dragging myself back to the bedroom.

Feeling sleepy. Maybe five more minutes of sleep couldn't hurt.

I reasoned that sleeping on amniotic sac fluid was less disgusting than sleeping in pee, so I made the lazy decision of fishing around in the dark for a new pair of underwear and a towel, rather than changing the sheets. After a quick change, I covered the wet spot on the bed with the towel and rolled on top of Damien like a sea lion on top of its mate. I nestled up and whispered in his ear, "Um, my water just broke."

Damien, who had been in a deep sleep, flipped me over as he sprang into a seated position. "*What?!* Are you *sure?!*"

"Yeah," I casually said. "At first I thought I peed the bed, but it doesn't smell like urine—so it must be my water."

"Do we need to go to the hospital, then?"

"Nah," I dismissed. "I don't feel any contractions or anything. Let's just go back to bed and we can go to the hospital in the morning."

This was music to his ears. He spun onto his side. Within seconds, he was twitching and snoring. It took me a little longer to fall asleep since, after all, we were going to be parents in the near future.

5:30 AM: I stirred and woke up. My head buzzed with excitement and I couldn't sleep any further. I hobbled to the living room and placed a towel underneath me as I sat down on the couch. I needed to be ready in case something unexpectedly came gushing out—like the elusive mucus plug!

Now that I think about it…where the hell is that mucus plug? Shouldn't

it have made its grand appearance by now? Please...tell me it's not floating around on the sheets!

I never did find that mysterious mucus plug. Ironically, as gross as
it may have sounded, I ended up feeling somewhat disappointed that
I never had a chance to see one up close.

I paged the doctor. All I could do was sit and wait in the dark for
her to return my call. I didn't feel or sense anything out of the ordinary, except a bit of leftover turkey coma from the prior day.

"I hope you're ready for this V."

*"Ready?! Are you kiddin' me?! I'm freaking out down here! Can't you
opt for a caesarean? I don't want no eight-pound gloppy monster sloshing
through me!"*

"Don't worry, V, we've got this! Well...hopefully one of us does."

At last...the phone rang: Dr. Decker.

"Karin?"

"Hi, Dr. Decker, yes it's me," I cheerfully answered. "How are you?
Did you have a good Thanksgiving?"

"Are you at still at home?" she demanded.

"Yeah," I replied through a yawn. "Damien and I were so wiped
out after yesterday. We made our first Thanksgiving for the family,
and—"

Dr. Decker interrupted me in an annoyed tone of voice: "Karin—
you *really need* to head to the hospital. *Right now.* Are you having
any contractions?"

"No, I don't think so," I considered, beginning to second-guess
myself.

Hmn. Maybe I am having contractions and just don't realize it?

"Okay," Dr. Decker exhaled. "You would definitely know it if you
were. Even so, you have to head over to the hospital—*immediately.*"

"Sure," I said. "I have to wake up Damien—"

"He's not awake yet?"

"—and I need a quick shower."

"*Karin*," she insisted. "You aren't understanding. You must come
in *right away.* Your water has been broken for a while, and we need

to monitor you. Grab your maternity bag and leave. I'll see you in the hospital."

Yeah. Right. There's no way I'm sporting amniotic fluid all day! Black Amethyst shower gel here I come. Never mind the embarrassment of having a bunch of doctors and nurses staring at my vagina's five o'clock shadow.

I put the phone down, patted Peanut on the head, and sauntered upstairs to wake up Damien and take a shower. When I was done, Damien hit the shower as well.

We went through our checklist for the hospital.

- ✔ Birth plan: *check.*
- ✔ Preggi Pops: *check.*
- ✔ Yoga ball: *check.*
- ✔ UNO cards in case I'm bored: *check.*
- ✔ Change of clothes for the baby and me: *check* and *check.*
- ✔ Surprise gift for Damien: *check.*
- ✔ V: *check.*

"Wait," Damien called to me. "Before we walk out the door, we need to take one last picture of you."

I struck a pose in front of the dining room wall that accentuated the profile of my belly.

"Smile!"

Damien snapped the pic, grabbed our items, and shouted: "Here goes nothing—baby time!"

To be continued....

THIRTY-TWO

A Totally Tear-able Surprise

OUR TALE RESUMES....

PARENTAL WARNING! Some of the graphic descriptions in this chapter may not be suitable for all readers—especially squeamish ones—without having a few drinks first (as long as you aren't currently pregnant).

The one thing no one tells a woman who is lying in a hospital bed waiting hours for the delivery process to commence: It can be excruciatingly boring. I'm talking boring, *boring*, B-O-R-I-N-G!

The arrival in the hospital was completely anticlimactic. I probably could've had even a few more winks, munched through a box of Ritz crackers, and painted my toenails before heading out.

Five hours dragged by. I admit I missed hearing from V, who had checked out and remained eerily silent throughout the entire day. I presumed she just had more important matters to tend to, or maybe she was silently cursing me.

With little to keep ourselves occupied, Damien and I played multiple games of UNO. Throughout our competitive card battle, I sucked on one Preggie Pop from among a variety of flavors after another. I was on fire, winning game after game.

If you don't know what Preggie Pops are, allow me to explain. Preggie Pops are essentially lollipops containing vitamin B6 that serve two purposes: curb morning sickness; and help prevent pregnant women from starving during delivery. I hate lollipops in general because they cause painful cuts in my tongue that linger for days.

So, why could I only eat these things? Apparently, someone made up a terrible rule that you can't eat before giving birth. This makes absolutely no sense, since plenty of women head into a last-minute labor after having wolfed down a plate of pasta or something spicy to induce labor, like chicken curry. Needless to say, I jumped on the lollipop bandwagon pretty quickly.

After a while, Damien became tired of losing at UNO and threw in the towel. Out of the corner of my eye, I spotted the yoga ball.

Ah—something else to do!

I didn't realize how much fun it was going to be bouncing on a yoga ball while dressed in a greenish hospital gown that could barely contain my butt. It was surprisingly comfortable as I checked work emails on my phone to inform everyone that I was going to be out for the foreseeable future. Periodically, nurses popped in to check my vitals and the numbers on the tape next to my bed. I stared at the printout to see if I could glean the baby's heart rate. I'm not a medical authority by any stretch of the imagination, but I knew that the bunch of crazy squiggles on the screen were better than a flat line.

One nurse, who was short in stature with a short brown bob, commanded the room whenever she entered. "How are you feeling?" she asked.

"Great!" I exclaimed. "Well, this gown isn't my shade of green—but, other than that, completely normal. This is nothing like in the movies at all." True enough, I was feeling pretty cocky. There were no debilitating contractions. I wasn't screaming at anyone. I was just my normal, bubbly self, waiting for a baby to arrive.

"Hmn," she said, looking back at the tape. "Well, let me know right away if that changes."

Sometime later, while I was in the zone bouncing on the yoga ball, Dr. Decker entered the room. She shuffled around the bed to the machine to study the tape. "So," she murmured with a puzzled look. "Have you felt any contractions yet?"

"Nope, nothing."

Her head tilted sideways.

That can't be good.

"Your body is having contractions," she informed me, dropping the tape. "Let's see how far dilated you are. Lie back for me. Put your rear at the end of the bed."

She patted the area where she wanted me to position myself and ventured down between my legs while snapping on a fresh pair of latex gloves. As I followed the instructions, Damien sidled up beside me. I shot him a severe look while motioning from the top of my body to my head. "Remember, you stay up here," I cautioned.

Dr. Decker chuckled. She'd heard all of this before. She inserted her hand—or maybe just a finger or two, I have no idea—into my vagina and retreated with an assessment: "Five centimeters dilated."

What's that mean?

A moment later, her head popped out from between my legs. "I think it's time to give you some Pitocin."

While my Mom didn't take an epidural, she was given Pitocin to help speed up the process, so I didn't think much of it. If there was anything to be concerned about, she most certainly would have told me. "Sure. Whatever you need to do."

"Shall I call the anesthesiologist in now?" she asked, though it sounded more like a command than a question.

I smugly waved her off. "No, I'm good. I'm going to try to make it without an epidural."

I peered over at Damien for reassurance. He smiled back with a look I interpreted at the time as saying, *"Wow—she's so brave and strong!"* In reality, though, he was probably thinking about what he was going to have for dinner in the hospital cafeteria.

Meanwhile, Dr. Decker gave me a look of her own that clearly communicated: *"Are you nuts?"*

I gave her a cavalier thumbs-up. She sighed, this time implying: *"You are totally nuts!"*

She administered the Pitocin. We thought something magical might instantly happen but, oddly, I didn't feel a thing.

Various nurses came and went to check my status. I asked each one what a contraction feels like and how I would know if I was having one. They all gave the same answer: "You'll know when you are having a contraction."

I didn't believe any of them since, apparently, I'd been having contractions for the past few hours and didn't know it. My cervix refused to dilate any further—even with the Pitocin.

"Karin," the doctor confided, drawing in close to me with her hand on my shoulder to indicate the seriousness of her message. "We're going to up the dose of Pitocin, so we can continue to attempt to move your labor along. Would you like me to call the anesthesiologist before we go ahead and do that? This is probably your last chance."

Hey, why do you keep asking me that? Look at me—I'm invincible! I don't feel pain! I don't need wimpy painkillers! I can do this on my own!

"I'm okay," I responded with a hint of irritation. "I got this!"

"All right, suit yourself."

The Pitocin was once again set into motion. Damien stood by my bedside, a real trouper. I prepared myself for another prolonged wait, realizing it might come down to a C-section.

There was nothing—until there was *something.*

"Whoa! Ugggghhhhh," I groaned, clasping my stomach.

What the fuck was that?

I looked to Damien for an answer, but his eyes remained trans-fixed on my belly as if an alien was going to pop out like in the Sigourney Weaver movies.

A minute later, after the crushing pressure subsided, I was struck by a revelation: I had officially been introduced to Mr. Contraction. I can't say I was pleased to meet him.

I shot Damien a look like I'd already been to hell and back: *You have no idea what that felt like.* I was about to voice the experience when, suddenly....

Uh-oh!

"Ow!" I howled, clutching my stomach to endure the onslaught. Damien tried to grab my hand, but I refused to move my hands. My vision began to fade in and out.

How am I going to get through this?

Just thinking about the next contraction added another layer of perspiration, as if I was running through a rain forest.

Not the makeup! I need to be camera ready.

One of the nurses suggested I try standing up and hunching over Damien's back. I don't know what gave her the idea that this had the slightest chance of working. In case you've forgotten, I'm vertically challenged, reaching 5'1" on a tall day. Damien stood about six feet tall. How on earth did she expect me to hunch over his back with my belly the size of a beach ball and only coming up to his butt? I'm not a mathematician, but even I know the proportions don't seem to add up.

Whatever—I'll try anything!

I wrenched myself out of bed and saddled up behind my husband. As my hands made their way over his shoulders, the next contraction hit.

Shitballs....

Words such as *shitballs* barely do justice to describing my agony. The closest I can come is saying it was like a hatchet tearing through my flesh. I could barely see through the black spots dancing in my eyes. Speech was out of the question. And—brace yourself for this— at the same time, I felt as if I had to drop a massive load (and I don't mean the baby).

What if I crap my gown? I'm not wearing underwear. It'll land right on the floor like that girl who pooped on Flavor Flav's reality show. I can't be like her!

The contraction passed. I collapsed in defeat. "Get me the anesthesiologist—and get him NOW!"

Dr. Decker reentered, flashing me a pleasant smile. I didn't interpret it as boastful or smiling in an *I told you so* way, but rather, as *Don't be too hard on yourself, most women end up caving.*

I would be lying if I didn't admit to experiencing some disappointment. I wasn't strong enough to make it on my own, which made me feel like I was letting women down all over the world.

Well, screw all that! So what—I'm not a hero. This is the birth of my baby. I want it to be a good memory.

The anesthesiologist was summoned. He ushered everyone out of the room. He issued instructions, which I followed to the letter. I hunched over the pillow and braced myself for the needle jabbing into my spine while using every ounce of willpower to remain still. I was convinced that, if I were to move a fraction of an inch, I would be paralyzed for life and never be able to hold my baby.

I didn't suffer for long. This anesthesiologist was my real superhero. He was done before I knew what hit me. "You'll be feeling better in no time," he assured me, bolting out of the room to his next patient.

Lo and behold, he was right! In a matter of minutes, I was one hundred percent numb. My legs turned to Jell-O, and I was back to cracking jokes.

I'm ready to have this baby!

Apparently, the kid wasn't as gung-ho as me, continuing to take his sweet time to make his grand entrance. Dr. Decker, who seemed eager to keep things moving along, directed me to start pushing. Now, if you've never had an epidural, here's what you need to know: It's like getting Novocain in your mouth at the dentist—multiplied by a thousand. In this case, instead of half of my face drooping, my entire lower half became useless. I couldn't bend my legs, which meant Damien had to hold my right leg while a nurse raised the left.

I delivered a final warning to Damien: "Eyes on me up here—or you're leaving."

"I know," he reassured me. "Now, get ready to push."

"*Push!*" the nurse roared.

This nurse meant business. I did as I was told. The only problem—I couldn't feel a damn thing, so I didn't have a clue how to push.

"*Push!!!*" she commanded.

Sir, yes sir!

I tried—I really did. I just didn't have the strength to figure this out. I was tired, starving, hormonal, and numb. Feeling the need to explain my failure, I shakily said, "I *am* pushing. I *think* I'm pushing. I mean, I'm *trying* to push."

"Come on, *dig deep!*" Nurse Ratched scolded me. "Take a deep breath and push that baby out!"

"*Aaaaahhhhh!!!!*" I yelled at the top of my lungs. While giving it my best effort, I imagined punching her in the face.

"There's the head," the nurse gestured.

At that moment, Damien did the unthinkable: He tried to sneak a peek at the baby's head.

Oh no—not going to happen, buddy.

My hand lashed out against his arm—a formal slap. His head jerked back.

That's right—back off! Try it again, mister, and you'll get far worse! If you see what's going on down there, you won't ever want to perform oral sex again.

Frickin' do this, Karin. If you shit, you shit. Just make it happen!

It took a few more all-out pushes before our beautiful baby boy emerged. They lifted him up. I laid my eyes on this tiny person for the first time. His arms and legs flailed about, but he was bluer than a blueberry. He hardly made a peep.

What's wrong with him?

The doctor promptly informed us there were two knots in the umbilical cord, which meant he'd been low on oxygen for some time.

"We need to rush him to the NICU—immediately!" she informed me.

"Can't I hold him first?" I begged.

"You have thirty seconds," she conceded.

Damien was permitted to cut the umbilical cord, while I stared into my little boy's eyes. He could barely open them, yet it seemed like he was looking right back at me. I fell in love with every little wrinkle on his face. I was terrified and overjoyed all at the same time.

Dr. Decker reached in and plucked him out of my arms. "We have to move, Karin."

Will I ever see him alive again?

And, like that, they whisked him off to an unknown location in the hospital. I was beyond worried, but not given any time to rest.

Here we go again…time for the afterbirth! Do I get paid overtime for this?

The grand finale is like the end of a Shakespeare tragedy: blood, gore, and guts everywhere. Yep, a big blob of red baby waste and undigested nutrients. The worst part: It's the same amount of work as the birthing process.

Take one guess what was next—cleanup time!

Nurses whizzed around the room removing equipment and sopping up anything that had spilled on the floor, leaving the door wide open—even though my birthing plan explicitly directed otherwise. I still didn't have any feeling from the waist down. Yet, I was thrown for a loop by Dr. Decker's cheery next statement: "Okay, Karin, I'm going to sew you up now."

"Oh no, I still plan on having more kids," I remarked, referring to having my tubes tied.

She didn't get the joke. "I know that. I mean, I am going to stitch up your tears."

"My *what?*"

"Honey, you tore quite a bit when the baby's head came through. I'm just going to get you stitched up. You won't feel a thing," she shrugged. "That epidural won't wear off for a while yet."

A second wave of sweat and anxiety swept over me.

Huh? I'm torn down there? That's it—game over. V is going to be off limits for months…maybe years!

Damien caught my petrified look, which caused him to react with equal concern.

Without warning, I unleashed the loudest, most rippling fart of my entire life directly in my doctor's face as she diligently sewed me up. Ever playing the "guy" role, Damien laughed out loud. I was mortified.

Someone. Anyone. Please. Suffocate me with my pillow.

I whacked him and barked, "You should be with our baby in the NICU. Get out of here."

He retreated out of the room, still laughing. I regretted having dismissed him so rudely after he'd stood by my side like a dedicated soldier through this whole ordeal for well over nine hours. I figured he'd have to understand, given everything I had endured.

My doctor, however, took it like a champ. She didn't laugh or flinch, just stayed focused on knitting poor V back together.

Before long, I found myself all alone in the hospital room. It was such an eerie feeling after all of the commotion and attention centered around me the past several hours. One would think I would've been happy to have a second to collect my thoughts and rest after just giving birth. Nope—it was quite the opposite. I wanted to see my baby, to know he was okay. I longed to see my husband and hold his hand. I wanted to go back to my prepregnancy, pre-torn body. Tears pooled in my eyes.

I was rescued by the doctor, who informed me we were moving to a different room for the remainder of our stay. All of a sudden, there was another flurry of activity as nurses made sure I was stable and in good shape, while orderlies began to straighten up. Although my legs were gradually coming back to life, they wheeled me into my new digs, where I tried to get comfortable in the hospital bed while waiting to properly introduce myself to my offspring.

When will they bring him to me? How is he doing after being deprived of oxygen? What if someone stole him and is escaping across the state border?

At last, it happened: Kyle—freshly cleaned, eggshell white, and swaddled in a blanket—was placed into my arms.

He's okay, after all. What a relief!

I gazed down, awestruck. He was the most beautiful thing I'd ever seen. All of my anguish, physical discomfort, and complaints went straight out the window. Damien joined us and we switched off holding him. Visiting hours were ending in thirty minutes, but I refused to let anyone else hold him—including our parents, who now paraded around the room—except the two of us. Everyone seemed to understand and be content with just gazing.

Everything was perfect. This was the longest I had gone in months without thinking about work. Not much mattered in those moments, except that a precious new life had been welcomed into the world. We were a happy, healthy family—the three of us.

As for V—well, she was an entirely different story.

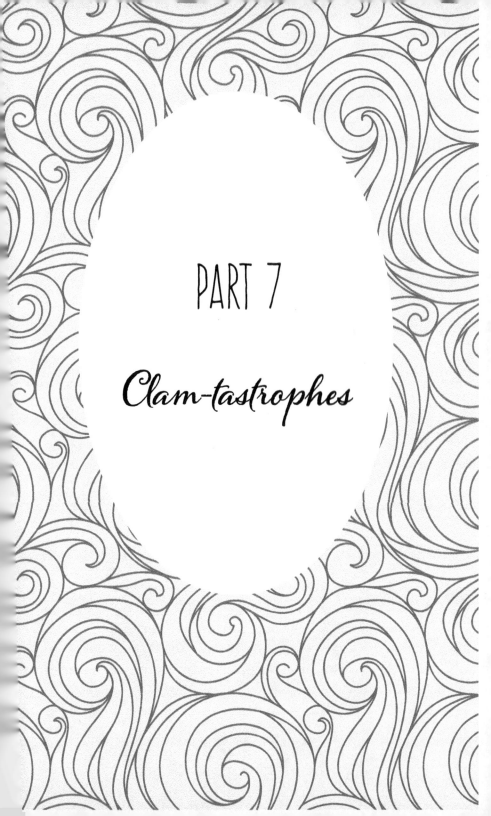

PART 7

Clam-tastrophes

$\mathcal{B}$y this point, in a span of almost thirty years, V and I had already been through a lot. We had conquered periods, yeast infections, and UTIs. We'd survived a miscarriage and brought life into the world. We had enjoyed good sex, bad sex, and a few world-rocking epic evenings. But nothing could come close to what we'd experienced in the days and weeks following childbirth. Any progress I might have made toward understanding my vagina and how it worked had been totally shattered.

Damn, I should have listened to my doctor and done more Kegels. Maybe, if I had strengthened my muscles, I would have been able to shove Kyle out in a way that didn't tear....

V and I weren't yet out of the woods—not by a long shot. As you'll soon discover, we had more trials and tribulations to face....

This is conclusive proof that guys have it way too easy when it comes to pregnancy and childbirth. They just hang out and watch, cut the umbilical cord, and get a snack from the cafeteria. They don't have to worry about a lazy penis that needs to be strengthened and worked out regularly or else it will turn into a limp question mark. Nor do they have to worry about their sex organ being mangled for an eternity. That's right, *an eternity*!

THIRTY-THREE

My Lamenting Labia

Is it a myth that all new parents become sleep-deprived zombies?

Nope. It's one hundred percent true.

The first week Damien and I were at home with Kyle was a mindless blur. Although my parents stayed over to help us out, Damien and I were awake and frantic pretty much all of the time. Breastfeeding couldn't have been more difficult. It's supposed to be a natural thing and a time of bonding between mother and child, but Kyle wasn't latching on and getting enough nutrients, which made it a frustrating experience for both of us.

Meanwhile, I was desperately trying to figure out how to pee without weeping. Thank goodness for the vagina numbing spray they gave me at the hospital! They even gifted me with an extra canister of the magical stuff to take home.

Okay, you're probably wondering if "vagina numbing spray" is a thing or if I just made it up as a joke. Trust me, it's *very real*! The idea is that you spray it on your vagina when the stitched areas hurt. For me, this was basically all the time, but exponentially worse when I sat down to pee with my vagina spread across the toilet seat. The pain was so great that I couldn't stand to look poor V in the eye. After urinating, I gingerly dabbed myself with some toilet paper and then liberally sprayed my tuna taco until feeling some semblance of relief.

"Ah, that's a lot better," V sighed. "Maybe you could lay off the coffee for a while, so we don't have the urge to go every twenty minutes!"

"Drink less coffee with a newborn? Have you lost your mind, V?" I blasted.

Eventually, I depleted my extra supply of vagina numbing spray, and was left without any relief for my encounters with the toilet seat.

Maybe I can get more on the black market?

After the first week or so, I finally summoned the courage to examine V with a hand mirror. I found the perfect opportunity: My parents had dashed out to grab lunch, Damien had returned to work, and Kyle was sleeping soundly in his bassinet. I had the house all to myself—which, as you should know by now, was usually when V and I got into trouble.

I locked myself in the bathroom, even though there was zero risk of anyone barging in. I pulled out my cosmetics hand mirror, took a deep breath, and stretched my neck downward.

"I don't know if you're ready for this," V warned.

"Why? How bad could it be? A couple of clean stitches, right?"

Wrong! Oh my God, the horror! The sight of V was worse than the goriest slasher film. She was unrecognizable, a mere shell of her former self. My right labia hung down like the roast beef lips I dreaded back when I was a teenager. The rest was swollen and stretched out, but at least seemed to be intact.

"V, WTF? How is our labia not sewn together? We're deformed!"

"Hey!" she protested. "I already feel bad enough. You're making me more self-conscious!"

The doctor had spent so much time sewing me up, she couldn't have just left my vagina lip like this.

Can this be fixed? Do I need reconstructive surgery? Will Damien ever want to give me oral sex again? What about the sensation down there— will it all be gone? Does it mean I will have unsensational sex for the rest of *my life? Will I have to tuck my labia into my thongs? This brings a whole new meaning to camel toe!*

My thoughts were interrupted by the sound of a crying baby. I wanted to cry, too, but I didn't have the time. The baby needed boob, *stat!* I stashed away my hand mirror, unlocked the door, and tended to Kyle.

I plopped on my bed with Kyle and whipped out my breast for him. Feeding time! Except...he wasn't eating. I made multiple attempts to reposition him, but they were futile. I couldn't figure out what I was doing wrong.

I was frustrated with my body from top to bottom—boobs, V, as well as everything above and in between.

My womanhood is being forced to retire and shoved on a dusty shelf.

I made up my mind to make an appointment with my doctor first thing the following day.

I can't deal with being the milk machine right now. You're getting a bottle!

Early the next day, I pumped plenty of milk for Kyle so I could leave him with my parents and set off to my doctor's office. As much as I didn't want to leave him when he was so young, I knew his grandparents could handle things and, more importantly, I needed to do this alone. I was too mentally distracted by my bodily woes to multitask with a baby in tow.

While in the waiting room, I was so preoccupied with repairing my ravaged lady garden that I couldn't bother to look at the magazines. Instead, I studied the other women who were in various stages (meaning, belly size) of pregnancy. I did not envy them one bit.

Guess what great stuff all of you have to look forward to. Should I warn them?...Nah!

The nurse called out my name. My vagina felt so raw and sore it took longer for me to get out of my seat and step across the room than when my tummy was housing a human life. I gave the nurse a fake smile when I finally reached her. She led me to an examination room and told me to undress from the waist down.

Déjà vu!

I stripped off everything except my socks. The room was freezing, and I couldn't imagine the doctor needed to see my feet anyway. Nothing says *sexy* like red wool socks covered in dog hair with a hole in the left heel and a postpartum body accentuated by a paper gown.

Upon entering the room, Dr. Decker flashed a warm smile and rested a hand on my shoulder. "So, what happened?" she asked.

"I don't know. I think my stitches came out. It's like my right labia is cut in half and now it's just hanging there like a broken shower curtain."

She grinned appreciatively as she began her examination. "Well, let me have a look."

I went into my usual position on the table and she went into hers. She rubbed her hands together before touching me. "My hands might be cold," she explained.

I felt a few pokes on my labia accompanied by concerned "hmn..." doctor-type sounds.

This can't be good.

Dr. Decker covered my body and stepped around the table to stand by my side. I could tell from her expression something was not right. I felt like a soldier in a World War II film being told a leg is about to be amputated.

No, doctor, please—leave the labia! I can tolerate the pain!

"What is it, doc? Give it to me straight."

"It does appear that your wound separated," Dr. Decker informed me.

Separated! Oh God, my life is ruined!

"YOUR life? What about ME?!" V gasped.

"The problem is that the skin has already healed," the doctor continued, "So, even if I successfully sew it back together, I can't guarantee it will stick."

My eyes become blurry. I started to feel faint. "What are my chances, doc?"

"It's worth a shot," she shrugged. "If it doesn't work, we could make a surface incision on both sides and then sew it back together."

"*Oh, hell no!*" V screamed.

This is the end. I can't do it. Go on without me. Just leave me here to die.

This was my worst nightmare: a future without any sex or, even worse, painful sex! The news, coupled with my post-pregnancy hormones, caused me to burst into tears.

"It'll be all right," Dr. Decker comforted me. "Let's start the procedure now."

Sew me up?! Here and now?! Will I have Novocain? Or another epidural?

Why did I listen to my mom and not get an episiotomy? It's all her fault I'm in this predicament.

"Can I at least get a six-pack of vagina spray to go?" I asked while wiping my cheeks. "I should have bought stock in that stuff."

This time, Dr. Decker couldn't resist chuckling. "You'll be fine, don't worry. I'll get the nurse to prep you for stitches. Just try to relax, it will only take a few minutes."

Relax? Yeah, sure. Easy for you to say. Give me a Corona and I'll find my beach.

My legs felt clammy. Sweat pooled on my upper lip. My body shivered.

A nurse entered carting a silver tray containing sewing materials and medical instruments.

Great, can't wait to share my hacked vagina with another person.

Dr. Decker entered while the nurse prepared her station and me for the procedure. Once again, I propped myself into position. "I'm just going to put some numbing cream on it," she said. "We'll let it soak in for a minute, so you won't feel it so much."

"*So much?*" I blurted.

"I'll be as gentle as possible," Dr. Decker assured me.

I tilted my head toward the ceiling and tossed myself a little pity party while she stitched me up like the Scarecrow from *The Wizard of Oz.* The nurse handed and removed instruments without making a sound.

Why me? Why V?!

"*Yeah, why ME?!*" V repeated.

"Ah!" V and I winced.

Guess what? The numbing cream doesn't completely numb you. It needs a new name, like *it still hurts like hell cream.*

"*Please, make her stop!*" V pleaded.

"*Stop?*" I replied to V. "*We can't have her stop. Then you'll be screwed up forever—and neither of us will ever get screwed again.*"

"You're doing great," Dr. Decker encouraged me. "Just a few more stitches and you'll be set."

"I just want to be fixed," I whimpered.

Several torturous minutes later...

"All done," Dr. Decker announced.

"Good as new?" I asked.

"Time will tell," she responded. "Let's hope for the best with the healing process."

Hope for the best? Is that all you can give me? Hope for the best?!

I bade Dr. Decker farewell. I made a mental note to update my birth plan. Getting the episiotomy was not only added on, it went straight to number one.

The days that followed were a time of great reflection. My vagina—every woman's vagina—is one of the things that defines her womanhood. (No two are alike.) Not only that, it's central to the creation of human life itself. Now there was a chance that my femininity was forever destroyed.

Will I be able to have sex again? Will I ever feel anything pleasurable down there? Or will it become agonizing and dry up forever like a fossil buried for a million years in the desert? Will Damien be repulsed by V?

Damien, V, and I would not discover the answers to these important questions for at least another five painful weeks. We could not take a chance on diving in too soon, as it would risk causing the stitches to pop open. For the time being, I had to live with my Frankenvagina and, well, hope for the best.

THIRTY-FOUR

Hot Dog in a Hallway

DAMIEN AND I NEVER THOUGHT THE DAY WOULD COME: THE END of our torturous six-week waiting period. While I rejoiced at having been cleared to have sex again, not all was positive news. The unthinkable happened: The labia stitches never took. V was doomed to be a cracked clam forever. Part of my womanhood sank into oblivion.

I was left with no room to sulk and mourn the loss of my perfectly shaped labia. Damien had been patiently waiting on the sidelines for a long time. Since I was given the green light, there was no way I could deny him at this point.

To be honest, I was as desperate as he was for some action. I can barely tolerate five days without sex, never mind six weeks.

I'd only had one brief encounter with my vibrator during the abstinence period, and the aftermath turned out to be a pretty upsetting experience. When I came out of my room after having satisfied myself, I checked on the baby in his bassinet and found him covered in spit-up. My first reaction was panic that he had nearly choked to death. My second was disgust with myself that he had nearly choked to death while I was playing the clitar. If word got out, everyone would have labeled me a bad mom, and I'd never be able to use a vibrator and orgasm again. Talk about traumatic!

Fortunately, Kyle was fine and only required a face wipe down. The experience taught me a valuable lesson, though: An awake child will never allow you to enjoy any kind of sex.

V, meanwhile, had mixed feelings. Part of her was raring to go, while the rest of her was terrified. Neither of us knew what to expect—pain or pleasure.

Damien peered around the kitchen door the instant I returned home from my doctor's appointment. "So...are we good to go?"

I yanked off my boots and responded, "Yep—she gave me the thumbs up."

"Sweet—"

"But—you gotta go easy on me!" I warned him. "None of that crazy jackhammer shit."

"I know, I know—don't worry. I'll be gentle, I promise."

He set a heated baby bottle on the counter and swooped in for a reassuring kiss.

We enjoyed dinner, after which Kyle went down for the night. Fun time! We figured we had somewhere in the neighborhood of three or four hours, which was way more than enough time considering Damien hadn't had the real thing in six weeks.

I snuck into our bedroom and made a quick change into my red baby doll outfit—the same lingerie I'd worn for him back in college. It was sexy, yet flowy and forgiving.

I don't have to worry about muffin top or back fat in this ensemble.

My hope was that he would only see the sexy young Karin he'd fallen in love with and forget about the rest.

I lit several candles along the wall and turned out the lights. I positioned myself on top of our fully made bed amongst the pillows, trying to channel my inner Tyra Banks and look as sexy as possible.

Come and get it, Big Daddy! Mama's ready for action....

"I'm going to vomit if you keep talking like that," V gagged.

"I think it's really sexy that he's a father now. Don't you?"

"I don't know, Karin. I'm so horny even Mr. Rogers would seem doable right now."

At that moment, milk began to leak from my right breast and soak through the push-up padding in my teddy. There was nothing I could do to stop it. The best I could hope for was to put my hand over my breast while twirling a strand of hair and pray he wouldn't notice.

Damien disrobed while trotting into the bedroom. He locked the door behind him, as if our newborn baby might barrel through at any moment and disturb our precious private Mommy and Daddy time.

We wasted no time exploring each other's bodies and doing all the things we hadn't been able to do in such a long time. He was understandably fixated on my swollen, milk-filled breasts, which I supposed was a good thing, rather than having him dive in between my legs where things were kind of murky.

Everything seemed to be going great, until...his mouth made its way to my nipple. This freaked me out, as I had been manufacturing lactose solely for Kyle's benefit—not his.

"You're getting uptight and killing the mood, Karin," V scolded.

"It's freaking weird, V. I'm like a cow. You don't suck on a cow's udders unless you're her calf."

"I don't even know what that means—but your man is getting his suck on right now and you need to get out of your head and back in the game!"

I tapped Damien's back.

He continued his activity with one eye looking up at me. "Hmn?"

"Can you taste the milk?" I asked.

"A little...it's kind of sweet. Why? Does this bother you?"

"No, no—does it bother you?"

"No, your breasts are amazing!"

He's going to be awfully disappointed when they shrivel up like raisins.

"Karin, can you shut up for two minutes?!" V exclaimed.

"You're right, you're right...."

Damien and I took our time with foreplay before getting to the main event. Aside from the weird boob conversation, we acted as if we hadn't missed a beat; at the same time, it was like we were making love for the first time.

Oh, how I missed this!

Damien took me by the hand and led me over to our rocking chair, which we only used when coaxing the baby to sleep. Clearly, he had another idea in mind for it.

"On the *rocker*?" I protested. "I feed the baby there."

"Come on. He won't know!"

"But *I* will."

"How many times have we had sex on the couch?" he countered. "You don't worry that my parents come over and sit on it all the time."

"Good point. Okay, fine."

He sat down and helped me climb aboard his naked body. The chair began to weave back and forth before we were in position.

Here we go...finally....

I easily slid down on his erect member. My mind was totally blown—but not in a good way. I felt nothing. *Absolutely* nothing. It felt like I was screwing a number two pencil that hadn't been sharpened. (Not that I would know this from personal experience.)

Oh my gosh, seriously? Did his penis shrink? What's happened to it? Maybe he lost his baby weight before I lost mine?

Then it dawned on me.

Duh...it must be that my vagina is all stretched out from having a baby. Oh no—I'm loose as a goose. I knew I should have done those damn Kegels like my doctor told me. Is this what sex is going to be like for the rest of my life? You could drive a Mack truck through V right now.

V did not care for my metaphor a single bit.

"Hey, I'm right here! I know all of your thoughts, remember? There's no need to be insulting, I'm doing my best!"

"Sorry...sorry...."

Meanwhile, I wasn't about to ruin things for Damien. He looked so ridiculously happy.

The one bright spot for me was that my labia didn't hurt. But it was a small consolation when I had lost all pleasurable sensation down there.

I resorted to making some fake passionate noises while continuing to glide up and down. What else could I do? He was so into it. I didn't want to hurt his feelings or skeeve him out. Luckily, my acting days had prepared me for this moment. Meg Ryan had nothing on me. He believed every second was authentic.

It didn't take long for him to climax. He felt accomplished and satisfied. I, on the other hand, felt depressed. We shifted over to the bed and snuggled under the covers in silence.

I can't believe he didn't notice anything...it was like putting a Tic-Tac in a whale's mouth.

I'll do whatever it takes—Kegels five times a day, every day. I'll do more foreplay, since the sex won't be good anymore. I'll consider vaginal reconstructive surgery. I'm sure it will be deemed medically necessary. They can fix my labia and tighten me up all at the same time. Yes—this is a solid plan: a comprehensive 100,000-mile tune-up.

I would conduct research on the procedures in the morning. In the meantime, I was emotionally drained and just wanted to put the whole evening behind me.

Damien leaned over my shoulder and kissed me good night. "I love you. I still think you're sexy," he reassured me. "Even if you haven't lost all the baby weight."

Ugh!

THIRTY-FIVE

Back in the Saddle

KEGELS, KEGELS, AND MORE KEGELS!

Kegels in the shower. Kegels while watching TV. Kegels during my commute to and from work. Kegels during breakfast, lunch, and dinner.

Something had to be done about my gaping vagina—and fast! You would have thought I was competing for the title of Woman's Strongest Vagina. This might even be a real thing. There are women who can shoot ping-pong balls out of their vaginas, as evidenced on an episode of *Tosh.0*. Talk about talent!

If you are among the women who haven't done the Kegel workout yet, you are probably wondering what it's all about. My doctor taught me the "elevator Kegel" method. I have no idea if there are different types of Kegels (like karate, with four main types: Goju-ryu, Shotokan-ryu, Wado-ryu, and Shito-ryu) or an "escalator Kegel." Here is how you do an elevator Kegel like a pro.

Don't forget to breathe the entire time you're doing your Kegels. It can be tough to remember, since you are so focused on counting and tightening. I admit I felt faint doing Kegels without breathing while driving my car, which is ill-advised when speeding on the highway.

THE KEGEL WORKOUT

*Picture an elevator in your mind.

1. Squeeze your vaginal muscles for five seconds. Be sure to breathe in and out; do not hold your breath.

2. During the five seconds, tighten the squeeze with increasing pressure until the elevator reaches the top floor.

3. Hold the elevator closed for a few seconds. This provides enough time for all the imaginary people to exit your vagina elevator. (You can say goodbye to them, if you wish.)

4. Gradually release your muscles, allowing the elevator to return to the ground floor to pick up some more passengers.

5. Repeat as many times in a row as your vagina can handle.

Often, I worried about whether anyone could detect that I was doing Kegels—especially when I was seated at my desk at work. The natural tendency is for your butt and stomach muscles to clench and flex along with the tightened vagina, which means other involuntary things are happening, too.

I wonder what my facial expressions look like to my colleagues while I'm riding up and down the Kegel elevator? Probably like I'm holding in a fart.

⑥⑨⑩

I continued to do the Kegel workout every day over the course of the next few months, even though Damien and I were way too exhausted to do much of anything outside parenting stuff, much less have sex. We went through all of the daily routines: feed baby; change diaper; read to baby; make breakfast; get ready for work; change diaper; drop baby off at daycare; try not to fall asleep and crash the car while driving to work; try not to fall asleep at work and get fired; pick up baby; return home; feed baby; change diaper; scarf down dinner; read to baby; give baby a bath; change diaper; go to sleep. You get the picture!

Since Damien was now an electrician and I didn't want him to electrocute himself as a result of being groggy and falling asleep on the job, we decided that I'd handle the night shift feedings Sunday through Thursday, while he would take care of them on weekend evenings. This didn't leave us much availability for intimate time.

One Friday evening, we decided we were overdue, and I believed V was in optimum shape for her Ironwoman competition. The plan was to start things off with a movie and a bottle of wine....

As soon as the baby went to sleep, Damien and I snapped into action. He dashed off to the liquor store for the booze, while I raced upstairs to slip on the perfect outfit.

"What do you feel like tonight, V?" I asked.

"How about some crotchless stockings and a black push-up bra?" she suggested.

"I can't watch a movie and drink wine in that! We need something sexy but more comfortable. I don't want you leaking all over the sofa, either."

"Good point!" she concurred. "What about the purple corset with the thigh-highs and garter belt. Can you deal with that for a few hours?"

"Definitely! I'll throw on some black heels for good measure."

I doused myself in some perfume—Miss Dior, his favorite. I curled up on the couch, wrapped myself in the largest blanket we owned, and waited for him to return. I was all revved up and ready to go. I just hoped he wouldn't come home too tired and reject me in my lingerie. There was a fifty-fifty chance of that happening, especially on a Friday.

At last, he returned. He didn't waste any time uncorking the bottle and filling two oversized glasses with pinot noir. He noticed I was bundled up in my blanket. "Are you cold?"

"A little—but between you and the wine, I'm sure I'll be plenty warm," I leered.

"Well, well," Damien crooned. "Looks like *someone* is in the mood tonight." He handed my glass to me and slid under the blanket while being careful not to spill his own drink.

In those milliseconds, he was able to get a good sense of my scanty outfit. "Are we even going to make it to the movie?" he smirked.

"I hope not!"

First things first. Let's get cozy.

We snuggled under the blanket and turned on the TV. Of all things, we chose to watch *The Simpsons* movie. Not exactly the most romantic choice, but at least it would be good for a laugh. Secretly I hoped Damien would be *eating my shorts* before the end of the flick. Damien and I had gone at it while watching far more unusual flicks in college, including *Ice Age*. (Maybe we had an animation theme going....)

Before long, we had downed our wine and were laughing our heads off. Damien dutifully rose, refilled our glasses, and returned under the blanket.

"Cheers," he toasted.

"Cheers," I replied, clinking his glass. We each took a nice long sip and then he made his move, swooping in for a long kiss. Four months of stress and exhaustion melted away. I hadn't felt this relaxed or sexy in ages. The kiss went on...and on...and on.

I can't remember the last time we kissed this passionately....

He repositioned the blanket on the couch and pushed me down on my back. He took his sweet time kissing me from head to toe. He hadn't made love to me this way in months—maybe even a year. It just hadn't been the same for either of us once my belly started to show.

I feel young, sexy, and in love again....

We switched off pleasuring each other. He gave me all the attention I'd been craving from the beginning of my pregnancy up until that moment. Since I was all dressed up—or was it down?—we weren't going to rush anything, and he refused to allow himself to finish early. Plus, this night called for something truly special.

"Stand up," he commanded.

I listened and rose from the couch, never breaking eye contact. He was in control and I loved every minute of it. It felt so refreshing for me to just live in the moment.

He spread the blanket out on the floor.

Wow—floor sex!

I obligingly went down on all fours.

This is it: the moment of truth. Will I feel anything?

I prayed to the Kegel gods as he slid inside me.

Please, don't doom me to pencil sex for the rest of my life.

V hooted like she had been cured of a grave illness at an evangelical event. "Woo-hoo! Thank you, Lord, thank you!"

"It's a miracle—it feels like a real penis again! Hallelujah! Can I get an amen, V?!"

"Amen, girl!" V rejoiced.

Everything was going to be just fine. My sex life was going to be fine. V was going to be fine, albeit slightly disfigured. I was on cloud nine—maybe ten.

I turned my neck around to get a look at Damien as he thrust himself into me with all of his might. I had to do a double take at his multitasking: While pumping, he was guzzling wine straight from the bottle.

Typical Damien!

I laughed out loud. He looked so hot and ridiculous at the same time. I was relieved to see that he was enjoying himself as much as I was.

"Want a sip?" he offered, extending the bottle out to me.

"Sure," I said.

He paused his motion so I could take a swig from the bottle without chipping a tooth and making a red mess all over the blanket.

"Thank you," I said, returning the bottle to him. "Please, proceed."

"Why are you being so polite to him during sex? We're not British royalty!" V mocked.

"Gotcha," I acknowledged.

"Give it to me harder, baby. Who's your dirty little slut?" I growled.

He gave it to me, all right. By the time he had finished, V and I were thoroughly pleased. Well—as pleased as any woman can be without having an orgasm.

At last, with confirmation that V had rebounded, Damien and I could once again enjoy sex. Of course, I loved him deeply throughout my pregnancy and during the postpartum months but, hey, let's face it, good sex is pretty darn important to a happy, sustainable relationship—for both parties.

I reluctantly admit that I got lazy after that and stopped my Kegel workouts. The elevator had gone up for the last time. Also, as I would soon discover, I had forgotten about one tiny but inevitable force…gravity!

THIRTY-SIX

We Have Liftoff

AFTER HAVING READ MY STORY UP UNTIL THIS POINT—AND PERHAPS having also heard far worse childbirth and postpartum nightmares—you are no doubt wondering why any woman would ever go through it all over again and attempt to have a second child. How soon we forget!

First, the miscarriage. Next, nine months of ballooning out and lack of sex. Then the interminable wait before excruciating labor. Followed by the agony afterward during the healing process. Plus, the gift of the torn labia. Not to mention the sleep deprivation.

And then...whoopee! One Friday evening, everything returns back to normal—except that Damien and I have a beautiful baby boy and my body is getting back into something resembling its former shape.

Baby number two? Why not! I'm ready!

Once my pregnancy amnesia firmly set in, I decided to casually broach the subject with Damien during dinner. Kyle was in a happy, cooperative mood, and I was able to strap him into his high chair and switch off between feeding him and myself. "Ya know," I began, giving Damien the eye glint that always stirred him. "It took a long time to get pregnant with Kyle. Maybe we should start trying for our second?"

Damien gagged on a mouthful of spaghetti while blurting, "A second?!" He swallowed and guzzled down some water before continuing in a calmer voice: "I don't know, Karin. Kyle's barely seven months."

I spooned some mashed peas into the baby's mouth, which he sucked right down.

"But Babe," I said, trying the logical approach with him. "If it takes us almost a year to get pregnant again, they'll be a good distance apart in age. I really want them to be close."

"I don't want them to be *too* close," he countered.

Kyle—looking very much like his father a couple of minutes earlier—spewed gooey peas all over his bib. I scraped the blob off with the spoon.

"You know our luck," I said, strengthening my eye glint. "It will probably take forever. I might as well at least go off the pill again."

"Okay," he relented. "I guess you could go off the pill and we'll see what happens."

"Great—I won't take my pill tonight," I confirmed, ensuring we were on the same page. Kyle was my only witness that we had agreed upon terms, but it would have to be good enough.

I was excited—and rather shocked—that Damien had caved so easily. My female superpowers clearly hadn't lost their force.

I stuffed more peas into Kyle's mouth, only to find them dribbling right back out.

"Want a hand there?" Damien asked.

Ugh. Why do I suck at feeding this kid? No one told me it was going to be this hard!

"No, I got it," I insisted, unwilling to admit defeat.

Eventually, I decided Kyle's body had received enough nutrition one way or the other, so Damien and I finished our meals and cleaned up the table. We settled the baby into his crib for the evening.

I sat on the couch with my iPad and began to scroll through work emails when Damien cozied up behind me.

"You look like you could use a back rub," he hummed in my ear.

"That would be *amazing*...."

He slid his hands up my shirt and unhooked my bra. He worked his strong hands into my neck and shoulder muscles. I didn't mind that his skin was somewhat callused from work. He had just the right touch, melting away a good portion of stress with just a few strokes. My eyes closed as thoughts of my work responsibilities faded away. His lips probed my neck....

Before I knew what hit me, he had positioning himself next to me on the couch and we were making out.

"Let's go upstairs," he whispered, rising to his feet.

"*What are you waiting for?!*" V snapped. "*The love train is leaving the station.*"

"*I have work to do,*" I pushed back.

"*Work?! You can do that later. His babymaker is primed and pumped— let's get busy!*"

"*I'm surprised you're so eager for a second child. What about all of the pain and suffering you went through the first time?*"

"*Pain? What pain?*"

All I could figure was that V's amnesia had settled in, too. I mindlessly followed Damien up the stairs toward our bedroom. We disrobed and initiated foreplay. We both enjoyed the gradual progression when he stunned me with a suggestion: "Go get your vibrator."

"What?"

"You heard me, don't play coy," he barked. "*Go get your vibrator.*"

Although we hadn't spoken about it in some time, Damien was well aware I still hadn't experienced the Big O with him. I thought he'd completely given up. Obviously, this was not the case.

"*Yeah, you heard him,*" V meowed. "*Get the vibrator!*"

"*I want to, V, I really do. But...I worry I'll hurt his feelings when he sees how quickly I'm able to get off.*"

"*Oh, give me a break,*" she dismissed. "*Like he's never been premature? This is your moment. Enjoy it!*"

I was torn. On the one hand, I longed to experience the pleasure I knew it would bring me; on the other, I was nervous and embarrassed.

Damien shoved me out of bed. "Go—I want to get you off!"

I couldn't believe what I was hearing. After so many years together, he still seemed so amenable to doing anything to help me become fully gratified during sex. As I made my way toward my dresser, I kept glancing back for reassurance that he was serious. He "shooed" at me to speed things up.

I sifted through my lingerie drawer in the dark. I'd never dreamed there was even a remote possibility of this happening, so I hadn't planned anything out.

Which one should I use? Maybe the one that seems least threatening to a guy?

With the above in mind, I opted for the egg-shaped, clitoral vibrator. I concealed it in my hand while making my way back to bed; I didn't want any chance of him seeing it and making any kind of comment that would spoil the moment. I placed the toy under the covers as I slid back into Damien's arms. To my chagrin—since I thought I would be the operator for the vibrator threesome—he snatched the device from within the sheets and deliberated on how to get it started.

Watching him fumble around made me impatient, so I cut to the chase. "You slide the dial up to increase the speed."

He followed my instruction, seemingly pleased to hear the toy produce a light buzzing sound. He placed it on my clitoris.

The effect of another person applying this to my body was immediate. I'm not exaggerating when I describe it as mind-blowing. My toes curled. My legs floated in the air.

I could sense that Damien was enjoying his newfound sense of power as he flipped me around on all fours and positioned himself behind me. This had always been his favorite position, but now he had the additional benefit of simultaneously stimulating me with the vibrator. He revved the dial to its highest setting before returning it to position.

"How does it feel?" he asked.

"It's perfect," I replied, reaching my arms back around his neck so we could kiss.

He plunged himself in as far as he could go. The pleasure enveloping my body from the combination of activity seemed like more than I could handle; it was so powerful that I had an instinct to stop by moving out of position.

Maybe I don't deserve it after all this time?

"*Speak for yourself, girlfriend! I, for one deserve this!*" V hollered.

"*I was talking to myself, not you,*" I said.

"*I don't care who you are talking to in your head—I hear everything!*" she shouted. "*Do not ruin this for me! Your man watched you give birth to your son. You created life with him. He loves you unconditionally. He also loves how you look and wants to please you. Don't take that away from him—or me!*"

"*You're right, V! But you better stop talking to me if you want this to happen,*" I remarked.

"*Copy that. Beaver over and out!*"

Each thrust sent shivers down my spine into my toes. I had no control over my body or mouth. My senses went on overload. In my mind, V assumed the form of a rocket ship about to take off. My pistons fired up. Smoke and flames jettisoned out of every pore. My arms released and the ship blasted off from the launch pad at warp speed. My body quaked. Somehow, amidst all of the tremors, I was able to summon enough inner peace to stay in the moment.

"Motherfucker! My pussy feels so good. Don't stop!"

Apparently, my trucker mouth was all it took for Damien to climax. Fortunately, my ship was already floating in the weightless ecstasy of space. Our baby making was off to a monumental start!

"*Holy shit, V! You did it! You finally had an orgasm during sex!*" I congratulated her.

"*Damn girl! That was...he was...I am—*"

"*Speechless! Who knew that was even possible!*"

Damien gasped for breath. "Did...you...get...off?"

"Yes! Is that what it's like for you every time?"

"Yeah! *Every time*," he emphasized.

"I'm so jealous. I want that every time, too!"

He laughed. "Well, at least now we know what you need."

"And now I know what *you* need!"

"Oh yeah, what's that?"

"Dirty talk!"

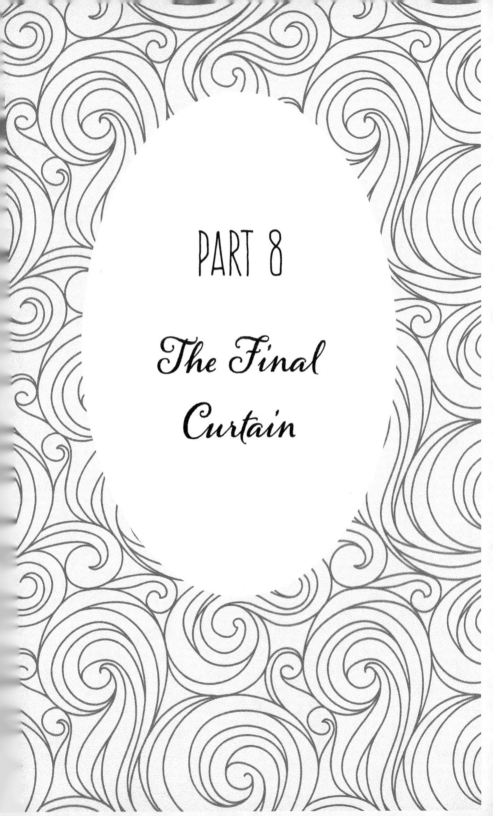

PART 8

The Final Curtain

$\mathcal{A}$ s I rose up in my company's ranks, I became a full-blown workaholic and everything else took a back seat to my career ambitions. We fit in the baby-making where we could, but V would still feel neglected when I was on a business trip or preparing for a work presentation. It's not that I didn't *want* to have sex more frequently; it just took too much time! When I did find a free moment, I would turn to my two-minute electric companions for immediate gratification. On the downside (as it were) it was also getting *really* expensive buying all those damn batteries for my toys! That is, when I wasn't stealing them from Damien and the kids. (Don't act like you've never taken them out of the TV remote or from your kid's toy in a dire situation. We've *all* done it!)

My hopes of a full-blown vaginal orgasm with Damien were fading further into the abyss. I had no illusions that I would ever be able to enjoy such pleasure without the aid of machinery. I know, many people have far worse problems than this, including life-threatening illnesses. But I'd spent the first three decades of my life longing for a vaginal orgasm. (Well, okay, maybe not quite that much, since I was closer to sixteen before I understood the concept.) And, let's face it, that's a long time to desperately crave something.

It wasn't just a physical desire. I longed for that human connection with my husband. I wanted him to be the cause to my effect. The yin to my yang. The hotdog to my bun. The cream to my cannoli.

Then there was my mom role, which can suck the romance out of any marriage. When you have a toddler, you're constantly covered in food, snot, and other bodily fluids. Not sexy! One thing they don't teach you in parenting class: *Your kids will never sleep, so you can kiss that hot, private sex good-bye.*

Are you jealous yet?

THIRTY-SEVEN

No Womb for Error

8:00 AM. I found myself in the bathroom at the doctor's office peeing into a cup. I had taken a home pregnancy test but the lines were blurry and I needed certainty. V was so enthusiastic that she nearly caused the cup to overflow. This was not a mess I was willing to deal with. I moved the cup out of the way just in time and completed my business. I wiped the sides of the cup with a paper towel, hoping no one would be the wiser.

The nurse was taken aback by the volume of my sample. "*Someone is well hydrated,*" she remarked, adding: "Head over to room five."

"Two cups of coffee will do that," I replied.

My phone buzzed incessantly from work-related emails and texts. I had an itch to answer them, but I had learned from experience that it was a bad idea for me to start getting involved in work stuff while in a doctor's office.

Three knocks on the door.

I could recognize those knuckle sounds anywhere.

"Come on in, Dr. Decker!" I shouted.

"Hi Karin," Dr. Decker merrily said as she swung through the door. "How's Kyle doing?"

"Oh, he's great. He's getting so heavy, I can barely carry him around anymore."

She laughed as she washed her hands. She dried her hands, straightened her glasses, and scanned my chart before turning to me. "So, it says here you are pregnant again? That was fast!"

"Yeah, we didn't really think it would happen so quickly but... surprise!"

"Let me examine your urine test results, which should be ready by now, and then we can celebrate. I'll be right back."

My phone seemed to be psychic, as it resumed buzzing the instant she stepped out.

It might be an emergency. Maybe I'll have time to answer one call....

The doctor came in just as I was about to cave and swipe my phone. I stuffed it back in my bag and watched her review my chart. "When was your last period?" she asked.

Why didn't she say congratulations? Something's up.

"I stopped the birth control sometime in August...I think I had a period in early September...maybe around the ninth? I think...."

"You're probably right at the beginning of the pregnancy," she deduced, looking up from the chart. "The urine test came back negative. Given you had a prior ectopic pregnancy, I think you need to go to the hospital right away and have an ultrasound. We need to be certain that the fetus isn't growing in your tubes again."

Are you serious? Another ectopic pregnancy? Am I going to need surgery this time?

"Do I need an appointment or anything?"

"No, I'll call over there now, so they'll be expecting you. You'll just go to the X-ray department when you arrive," she instructed. "We'll talk about next steps once we know the results of the ultrasound."

She placed a reassuring arm on my shoulder. We'd been down this road before and I had every confidence she'd figure it out.

I held off filling Damien in on my situation. Why bother him when I didn't have all the facts? Instead, I turned off my phone. I'd arrived at my destination and didn't want any chance of a distraction—not when the stakes were this high.

A few minutes later, a nurse led me to a dark, cold room for my ultrasound. She handed a gown to me and ordered, "Everything off and open in the front. The technician will knock before she enters."

I nodded yes, unable to muster a smile. This feeling was all too familiar. I had an intense flashback to being at NYU getting the ultrasound to confirm my miscarriage. I undressed and situated myself on the table next to the machine, which made a soft humming sound much like white noise.

The technician entered. She was skinny and filled the room with the aroma of stale cigarette smoke. The back of her dusty brown hair was tied up in a sloppy bun, while her unevenly cut bangs fell over her eyes.

I hope she reads ultrasounds better than she manages her hair.

Since it was so early in the pregnancy, she had to use the wand to examine inside my vagina. She wrapped a condom over it, presumably to prevent the spread of germs. She inserted the cold device inside of me and proceeded to move it around in different directions.

"Man, this thing feels awful!" V cried.

I ignored her bellyaching to concentrate on the technician's actions. Once she had a position and angle that seemed just right, she clicked on her keyboard to take pictures.

"Should I say 'Cheese'?" V remarked.

I drowned V out in my head by questioning the technician. "What is it? Are you able to see anything?"

She chose her words carefully before responding. "No, not yet. There is something in one of your ovaries—but it might be a burst cyst. It's hard to say."

I know what this means. I'm probably going to have another ectopic pregnancy.

My hormones were out of whack from recently going off birth control. To prevent myself from breaking down into an emotional mess, I squinted at the monitor in a desperate attempt to detect a baby where the technician couldn't.

She read through my chart again. "From the notes, it looks like you had your period in early September. So, you're probably only about three weeks pregnant."

I didn't know what to make of that comment, other than perhaps it was just too early to see anything on an ultrasound. I knew what was next if they couldn't find the fetus: *laparoscopic surgery*.

She extracted the wand and handed over a white towel to clean off the lubrication.

"What, we don't get a cigarette?" V joked. *"She must have an extra in her pocket."*

"Stop," I berated. *"This is serious."*

"I told you I thought it was too soon for us to put a baby in my oven again. Just when we were finally getting the Big O with Damien!"

"Shut up, already!"

I got dressed and returned to the waiting room, where I found a seat in the corner as far away from other people as possible. I turned on my phone for only one reason: text an update to Damien.

> Bad news, Babe. I'm at the hospital. Doc thinks it might be another ectopic pregnancy. Will call when I know more...

The doctor, a scrawny man with black-framed glasses and a prominent bald spot on his head, summoned me into an exam room. "I'm Dr. Schwartz," he introduced himself. "I've reviewed your results. At this stage, we believe the fetus is stuck in the fallopian tube. It is our recommendation to terminate the pregnancy to ensure you are safe. Ectopic pregnancies are very dangerous for the mother."

"I don't understand," I blurted. "The technician said it could just be a cyst that burst."

"Well, we don't know anything for certain," he clarified. "However, since we can't see the egg implanted anywhere else in your uterus, it leads us to believe that the pregnancy is in the tube."

I sobbed for a couple of seconds before stating, "I want to call my OB."

"Yes, of course. We'll give you a minute," he said, stepping out of the room.

The tears flowed freely.

Why won't these eggs go to the uterus like they are supposed to? Is it because of the birth control? Should we have waited longer before trying? What is wrong with me? What is wrong with my vagina?

"*Hey, don't blame me!*" V protested. "*I can't control it!*"

I pulled myself together enough to make my call. The receptionist answered on the first ring. "Dr. Decker's office, how may I help you?"

"Hi, this is Karin Freeland, a patient of Dr. Decker's," I began, taking a deep breath. "I was there just this morning and I'm at the hospital for the tests she ordered...."

Don't cry, don't cry...hold it in...

Nope. I could not hold it in. "*I neeeeeeeeed to speeeeeeaaaaaak with heeeeeeeeer—please!*" I wailed. I took another deep breath before continuing. "I'm sorry, I received...bad news."

"Oh yes, honey," the receptionist said with convincing sympathy. "One sec, I'll run and grab her."

Hold music piped into my ears for a few seconds until Dr. Decker's reassuring voice came on. "Karin?"

"Yes, I'm at the hospital," I sniffled.

"What did they say?" she asked.

"Well, they want me to have the surgery today," I informed her. "But I don't want to do it. I'm afraid. What if they're wrong? The technician said she wasn't even sure if it was a fetus or a burst cyst."

"Can you have them email me a copy of the results?" she suggested. "I want to take a look. We aren't going to do anything until you are comfortable."

Dr. Decker to the rescue!

"I'll ask. Hold on."

I poked my head out the door to see if I could find someone to provide what Dr. Decker required. I signaled to a nurse who was passing by. "Can you please send my ultrasound results to my doctor right away so she could look at them now?"

"Sure, we just need her email address," the nurse complied.

I provided both sides with the necessary information, hung up the phone, and called Damien. Texts weren't going to cut it.

He answered right away. "Hi, what's going on?"

"Did you see my text?"

"No, sorry. We're on a big pipe run today…."

"The pregnancy test at Dr. Decker's office came back negative, so they sent me to the hospital for an ultrasound."

"And?"

"They're telling me to have surgery to abort the pregnancy," I said. "But I'm scared. What if they are wrong? What if it's *not* ectopic? I just have this feeling. The technician said one thing and the doctor is saying something else. I don't want to do it."

"So *don't*," he asserted. "Can you wait?"

"A little while," I answered. "Dr. Decker is reviewing the ultrasound. I'll have to hang up on you when she calls."

"If you don't know, don't do anything," Damien commanded.

Thank God for Damien. He's supportive, as always.

"They're worried I could pass out or die if it really is ectopic," I said. "But I would have symptoms, so I guess I could just come back if I have bleeding…."

Another call came in. I knew who it was without even looking. "Gotta go, she's calling me. Keep you posted."

Click. I switched to the incoming call.

"Karin?" Dr. Decker asked.

"Yes, it's me."

"I just had a look at the ultrasound images. I *agree* with you. It's not conclusive enough at this point," she proclaimed. "I think we should wait before doing anything."

What a relief.

"But listen to me," she sharply continued, "If you have *one* stomach cramp, one minor abdominal pain, or one drop of blood, I want you back in that ER immediately. Do you understand me? This is life or death."

"Yes, I do," I agreed. "I promise, I will. Thank you so much."

Later, when Kyle arrived home from daycare, I hugged him a bit tighter than normal. It felt good, but it also made me worry even more.

What if it really is ectopic? What if I never get to hug my baby? Normally, a drink would be just the right pick-me-up, but I'll have to settle for drowning my sorrows in a huge bowl of vanilla ice cream with chocolate sauce.

The next few days, I was a complete neurotic mess. I checked myself from making any potentially reckless moves. I inspected every inch of my body throughout the day to be on the lookout for any aches, pains, or swollen breasts. I started taking prenatal vitamins. I even threw in an extra prayer at night. I hardly slept a wink.

The week seemed like it would never pass but, finally, it did, and I found myself once again in Dr. Decker's office taking a pregnancy test. This time, the results came back *positive*. While it was an important piece of information, it didn't reveal whether the pregnancy was ectopic or not.

Déjà vu: back to the hospital for an ultrasound. The same technician with the bad hair, the same cigarette smell, the same exact procedure.

Silence. Followed by more silence. She took the picture and brushed a clump of hair away from one eye. "I can see the fetus," she said, gesturing to the screen. "It's right here in your uterus."

I peered over but couldn't discern a thing. I'd have to take her word for it. Either way, it was music to my ears.

We're having a baby, after all—and I'm not going to die!

My first reaction was to want to jump around and do a happy dance. I didn't, however, because a moment later I began to feel irate.

Didn't that Dr. Schwartz suggest surgery and termination of the pregnancy a week ago? How could he get this so wrong? What if I'd listened to him? My baby would never have a chance to be born. Thank heaven for Dr. Decker!

I called Damien right away and breathlessly told him, "We're pregnant! It's all good, not ectopic!"

"That's awesome! What's the due date?"

"June ninth," I replied. "I'm so glad I won't have to be pregnant all summer. But don't tell anyone until I'm three months."

"I know, I won't. Well, I'll see you when I get home."

"Sounds good. Love you," I said.

"Love you, too."

"Thank you, V! Thank you for not screwing this up for us."

"You owe me big time for this!"

"What do you have in mind?"

"Let's just say it involves a pair of thigh high stockings, a full-length mirror, and Damien's secret weapon. Oh—and no baby bump!"

THIRTY-EIGHT

Sex + Pregnancy = Catastrophe

PREGNANCY NUMBER TWO DIDN'T HINDER OUR SEXUAL DRIVE OR activity—at least not at first. Why not? It was all gravy! It was too early to detect any sign of a belly bump and round ligament pain wasn't even a blip on my radar. Plus, I had those giant, luscious breasts, which were a gift for both of us. I felt like a porn star with my new knockers (or "seasonal fruit" as Damien always referred to them). It was *all* good! We didn't have a care in the world and the sex was fun. Even exhaustion from chasing around a toddler couldn't discourage us.

But then...the party abruptly ended. My belly bulged, and it was all over for my body. By the third month, I was in maternity pants; after six months, my womb became officially possessed by an alien. Both of my boys were jiujitsu masters while gestating. I'd be sitting at work and suddenly an elbow, fist, or foot would go ripping across my stomach, as if the lining were a concrete block meant to be split apart. Imagine trying to have sex while that is happening—it's a wee bit challenging to stay in the moment.

Damien was also one of those guys who didn't find me as sexy when I was pregnant. I can't say I blamed him. I wouldn't have wanted to screw me, either, with my bump turning into an oblong beach ball. More than that, though, he was just kind of freaked out that there was something living in my belly and he didn't want to hurt the baby. Being a guy, however, he still had his needs.

One Saturday night, I dressed up in a hot pink silk teddy with matching thongs from Victoria's Secret. It wasn't see-through, as the whole point was to hide my bump as much as possible. It had a big silk bow over the chest of the teddy, which accentuated my breasts even more. It made me feel special and, considering most weeknights we didn't have the time or energy for that type of fanfare, it put me in the mood.

Since I couldn't position myself in a sexy way on the bed in my condition, I leaned against the bedroom doorway and struck a pose. "Damien," I called downstairs. "Can you come up here? I want to show you something."

He took his sweet-ass time getting up the stairs. I felt like I was standing in that stupid flamingo position forever. Finally, he made it to the top of the landing, rounded the corner, and spotted me waiting for him. He shot me a boyish smile while breathing me in.

"Is this new?" he asked, running his hands along the back of my silk teddy.

"Yes, I just got it last week," I leered. "Do you like it?"

"It's nice," he said, flicking the lights.

"I don't know, V. Maybe we should abort the mission."

"Don't even say that!" she recoiled. *"The way your belly is growing, it's now or never!"*

I stood up on my tippy-toes to kiss him, but my stomach bounced into his like Jell-O. We laughed. What else could we do?

He led me toward the bed, where I helped him remove his clothes before he perched himself at the edge. This only meant one thing: *blow job.*

I flopped onto my knees to get into position. I leaned forward when something got in the way: my stomach. My mouth was miles away from his penis. I'd need the neck and tongue of a giraffe to reach him.

"Move closer to the edge of the bed," I instructed.

He shifted over as I suggested. Feeling somewhat humiliated, I closed my eyes and went to work.

During both pregnancies, I found it difficult to catch my breath while exerting myself with pretty much any activity. All of the up and down with my head provided limited air intake for my lungs. It didn't take long for me to become winded.

"I can't take much more of this, V. Can you imagine if the baby and I die from lack of oxygen?"

"You better stop," she warned. *"You don't want the cause of death to be blow job—that would be pretty embarrassing for everyone."*

"Agreed—that would be no bueno!"

Sensing my struggle, Damien tapped me out.

Gracias, papi.

He made it clear that we weren't nearly done—but we both knew our options were limited to two: wiggly worm (spooning with him behind me) or doggystyle. In both cases, he could enter me without the bump getting in the way and use his hands to take advantage of my enormous breasts.

We assumed one of the positions and got busy. It went along fine for both of us until he climaxed. I admit, it was something of relief. I was breathing so heavily that in another couple of minutes I would have been hyperventilating.

"I can't wait…to have my body back to normal," I huffed, fishing for a compliment.

"Just don't lose those breasts," he said, remaining inside me throughout our conversation.

It wasn't exactly the compliment I'd been searching for, but I played along with him while also interested in getting his thoughts on the subject. "I could get implants. What do you think?"

"No," he stated. "You have a family history of breast cancer and implants can make it harder to detect. I just love them when you're pregnant. Your normal boobs are perfect."

Good point. Impressive.

An itch on my stomach chose that moment to flare up. I'd noticed the condition earlier in the week and assumed the skin had become dry from all the skin stretching.

I nudged Damien to hand over some paper towels, so I could get up and find the moisturizer without making a mess from V. He placed the roll in my hands. We coordinated his withdrawal from me in such a way that I could catch his fluid with the towels. He used a few more sheets to clean himself off.

"Whoa, Karin, you're bleeding," he observed, jumping out of the bed.

"I am? How much?"

"Like—*a lot.*"

He turned on the light. We both stared in horror at the bright red splotches on the paper towels in his hand.

"Oh, shit!" I exclaimed.

My attempt to sit up with my pregnant belly was a total failure, as I got stuck in the memory foam of our bed. Damien grabbed me by the elbow to help hoist me up. I hobbled to the bathroom, where I plopped down on the seat.

Oh yeah, there's a lot of blood in there.

Panic set in right away. I'd never experienced this with Kyle's pregnancy. I could hear Damien pacing in the hallway as I cleaned myself up, threw on a pantyliner, and got dressed.

"Should you call the doctor? Do you think we should go to the hospital?" he asked the instant I appeared out the door.

"I don't know," I replied. "I guess I should try the doctor on call and see what she thinks. My stomach is starting to hurt—kind of where my ovaries are."

A minute later, I was sitting up in my bed listening to the answering service operator. "How can we help you?"

"Hi, I'm a patient of Dr. Decker's, and I just had sex with my husband," I babbled. "Now I'm having some bleeding and I'm worried. I'm also having some pain in my abdomen around my ovaries. Can you ask one of the doctors to call me?"

"Sure, Dr. Nola is on call…."

Ugh—it figures that one of the male doctors is on call tonight. He's the last person I want to talk to. It's just awkward. Ten minutes ago, my husband was nailing me good—and now I'm bleeding. He'll probably think: "What kind of husband is so rough with his pregnant wife?"

The pain intensified during my wait for the doctor to return my call. I broke into a sweat as I doubled over clutching my stomach.

Please, don't let anything be wrong with the baby!

This reminded me of the pain I'd experienced when I was younger. I would've been willing to bet it was an ovarian cyst that had popped and ruptured—but I needed to be certain.

My phone rang a few moments later. My heart pounded. "This is Karin."

"Yes, hello. This is Dr. Nola. What's going on?"

"Hi doctor. Well, I'm a few months pregnant and…my husband and I just had…*sex*," I said, sounding like a guilty teenager. "Um… afterwards, we noticed a lot of blood. I'm also having sharp pains in what feels like my ovaries. I'm scared for the baby."

"No problem. It's always best to call when you have questions. How long ago did you have sex?"

"I think he lasted about forty-five minutes."

"No, no, no. I meant how long *ago*."

Somehow, I missed hearing one important word: *ago*.

I'm such a ditz.

"Oh, geez, right. About twenty minutes ago," I answered.

"I see. Are you still bleeding?"

"I just went to the bathroom and, yes—but there was less than before."

"Okay," he absorbed. "I think you just bothered the lining. This can happen when you have sex during pregnancy. But don't worry, I don't believe you hurt the baby."

"What about the pain? It was really intense after we had sex."

"Do you have a history of ovarian cysts?"

"Yes."

"That's most likely what it was. Lay down and rest a bit. If the pain persists into the morning, call me back. Okay?"

"Okay."

Sure enough, the pain and blood subsided the following morning. False alarm. The only thing damaged was my pride.

"*You mean—our pride*," V corrected.

"*Whatever*," I countered.

"*So*," she continued, trying to summon the right words. "*You aren't thinking about closing up my shop, are you?*"

"*Not on your life*," I snapped.

"*Phew*," she sighed in relief.

"*But we're going to have to be extra careful. I'm not going through this again*," I reprimanded. "*You get what you get, and you don't get upset.*"

"*Don't pull your parenting crap on me! I don't really care...I don't need sex anyway.*"

"*Nice try using reverse psychology! Who's acting like the parent now?*"

THIRTY-NINE

The Levee Breaks

IT WAS A TYPICAL SUMMER SUNDAY MORNING. KYLE WOKE UP AROUND 5:00 AM for his bottle. I struggled to keep up with him as he toddled around the house, leaving a path of toys in his wake.

What I wouldn't give for an iced coffee....

I felt like my baby was going to drop any moment, even though it was four days ahead of schedule. I half-expected to see an arm dangle out from between my legs and start waving at me.

After a while, I decided I couldn't stand another minute without a shower, so I plopped Kyle on Damien, who was still fast asleep. "Good morning!" we both shouted at him.

Damien groaned with his eyes remaining shut, but I didn't have any patience. "Watch Kyle," I ordered. "I'm hopping in the shower."

My stomach started itching as soon as the hot water hit my body. While scratching myself, I noticed a sea of red markings had formed around the bottom of my belly.

I had been terrible about applying cocoa butter the second time around, thinking I wouldn't have an issue. After all, I was a pregnancy pro, right?

I lathered up with my loofah, intermittently digging my nails into my skin. I exited the shower, dried myself off, and spread cocoa butter all over my belly as a precaution.

On my way downstairs to rejoin Damien and Kyle, I felt a twinge.

"Did you feel that?" V inquired.

"Yeah, do ya think it's what I think it is?"

"I'm not ready—it's way too soon!"

"It's definitely not too soon," I admonished. *"And don't you dare go trying to hold this thing in. We need this baby out—now!"*

"Maybe we have time to squeeze in one last romp?"

"I wish—but we're not going to the hospital to deliver a baby with semen dripping out of us, thank you very much."

I mentioned the sensation in passing to Damien—just in case.

He headed straight into panic mode. "Did your water break yet?!"

"Does it *look* like my water broke?" I chuckled.

Then again...I was in the shower, so I don't really know.

"I'm just going to lie down on the couch," I said. The situation was starting to become real.

"Make sure to put a towel down, Karin. I don't know if you can get amniotic fluid out of microfiber."

I probably should have felt insulted by the remark; however, I realized he was most likely right and positioned a towel on the couch before my body took over the length of it. It only took a few more pangs accompanied by tightness in my stomach to tip me off that something was genuinely happening, and I needed to call the doctor's answering service. Once again, I was informed that Dr. Decker wasn't on call that weekend; the doctor wasn't even an OB-GYN from my practice. This time, at least, the doctor was a woman. She suggested I get checked out at the hospital. She seemed friendly but, female or not, I was nervous about being treated by an unfamiliar doctor. Thankfully, Damien and I were prepared with our birth plan in hand.

On our way to the hospital, we dropped Kyle off with friends. When we reached the hospital, Damien parked the car in the visitor lot. In hindsight, he probably should have pulled up to the curb so I could slide into a wheelchair, but I figured the walk might do me some good. My biggest gripe was that my stomach itch flared up again. I blamed it on those stupid (yet necessary) elastic waist bands all maternity pants and shorts seemed to have. I snuck in scratches as we made our way through the parking lot, onto the curb, through the automatic door, and up to the reception desk.

Once the paperwork was filled out, I was escorted via wheelchair into a room where the nurse provided me with the typical unfashionable gown. Two minutes later, the most beautiful woman I'd ever seen entered. She had gorgeous dark brown skin and her hair and makeup were Hollywood perfect.

"Hi, I'm Dr. Diane Jackson," she beamed, extending her hand to me for a shake. Her nails were expertly manicured, and her hands felt soft and supple. I was so in awe of her—and acutely aware of my own frumpiness—that all I heard was "Dr. Diane."

If Dr. Diane is as talented a doctor as she is beautiful, we're going to be all right!

I didn't waste any time handing her my birth plan and expressing my foremost thought: "Dr. Diane—whatever happens, just make sure I get the episiotomy!"

She glanced at the piece of paper before tucking it into my chart folder. "We'll try our best," she said.

I needed a lot more reassurance than that. "Seriously, Dr. Diane, I don't want to tear ten ways to Sunday like last time—just cut me, okay! Do whatever you have to do to keep me intact."

"Sure—but one thing at a time. Lie down on the bed. Let's see how far you've dilated."

She snapped on a white latex glove while I got into position. When we were both ready, she began her examination.

"You're about four centimeters—definitely in labor," she concluded. "Your water hasn't broken yet, so we may have to break it for you. I'll be back in a little bit to check on you."

When Dr. Diane left, I suggested to Damien that he phone our parents, figuring we were in for the long haul. He conveyed the details, hung up, and turned to me. "My parents are on their way. They'll go to the house with Kyle and wait for us to call when Ricky is born."

Ricky—what a nice ring!

Since waiting was all we had to do at this point, I proactively requested the epidural. I'd learned my lesson the last time around. There was zero need for me to experience all that pain again!

The anesthesiologist harpooned me with the needle, and I entered my happy place, good and numb. Like Dr. Decker during my first labor, Dr. Diane seemed anxious to keep things moving, so she broke my water.

The hours passed without incident, during which time I was forbidden to eat a thing. I became so starved as evening set in that I snuck Preggie Pops—which I had left over from Kyle's birth—when medical personnel weren't around.

Another four hours limped by. Damien fell asleep in a chair next to the door. Bored, I flipped through work emails. Finally, at around 11:00 PM, Ricky made his move. The deathly still room became energized with activity: Dr. Diane, nurses, and orderlies went to work, shining a spotlight on V.

"*All eyes on me,*" V chanted whimsically.

"*This isn't a Tupac concert, V!*"

Damien abided by the rules, positioning himself near my head. Dr. Diane worked her magic down there—whatever that entailed— while I pushed for a good hour straight.

A head suddenly popped out—Dr. Diane's, that is. "Karin," she forcefully said. "The baby's head is about to come through. I'm going to make a small incision in the rear of your vagina."

"*No—please, don't!*" wailed V.

"We have no choice—the alternative is worse!"

"Cut away!" I authorized the doctor.

I death-gripped Damien's hand for a surge of final superhuman pushes until we heard the cries of our baby boy entering the world.

Nothing could have sounded sweeter. Plus, unlike the last time, there were no complications.

Time to pop the champagne bottle—I deserve it!

It was too late to receive any visitors, so Damien and I enjoyed our private room in peace and quiet. Once examined, weighed, hosed off, and bundled up, baby Ricky was returned to us, fresh and clean—all seven pounds, eleven ounces of him.

Wow, I'm a parent of two!

Damien conked out in his chair, while Ricky slept peacefully in a baby bassinet, which was more like a plastic bin. I needed a good doze myself, but I desperately had to pee.

Fortunately, the feeling had returned to my legs, so I was able to swing them off the side of the bed and get to my feet. I made my way to the bathroom with caution, less because I didn't want to wake anyone than due to soreness from the delivery.

I flicked on the light and tugged down my black maternity yoga pants and underwear. I clasped on to the gray metal railing as I lowered myself to the seat.

I guess these aren't only meant for old people....

"Yowza!" V and I exclaimed in unison.

Every inch of my nether regions was seared in agonizing pain. I vowed not to drink another sip of anything—even water—until I was completely healed. Gross as it may seem, wiping was out of the question; the best I could do was a light dab. Then something caught my eye—the *good stuff*. The mother of all pain relievers. My old friend, vagina numbing spray.

I wish I could find the person who invented this and give him or her a big hug.

I went on autopilot for the remainder of the night with feedings and diaper changes. A nurse came in to check on me and the baby around 7:00 AM.

"Good morning, Karin," chimed the bubbly nurse as she opened the shades, which blinded me with sunlight.

"Morning," I droned.

"How did you sleep?" she asked.

"Um...something in the vicinity of *none*? I'm not sure if he's getting enough to eat."

"Would you like me to send in the lactation consultant?"

"Yeah, that would be good."

"Have you gone to the bathroom yet?"

"Yeah, I went once last night."

"Only *once*? You better drink some more water, so you don't get dehydrated."

"No thanks. It hurts too much."

"Well, if you aren't hydrated, you are going to have a harder time breastfeeding."

Damn it! She has a point.

"I guess I need some water then," I relented.

She grabbed my pitcher and began to fill it up when Damien stirred in his seat. "By the way," she addressed Damien. "You better help out—your wife looks like shit."

Whoa! Did she just say I look like "shit"? Do I look that bad? Perhaps a touch-up is in order.

I grabbed my makeup bag off the side table and pulled out a mirror. I took a long, hard look at my face.

I do look like shit.

My face was gaunt and my skin pale. The bags under my eyes looked like duffels packed for a lengthy trip. My greasy bangs stuck to my forehead.

Damien, still feeling the sting of the nurse's comment, sprang out of his chair and asked what he could do to help.

"How about growing a pair of tits and feeding Ricky?"

He played along like a good sport. "Sorry, can't do that."

"Yeah, I didn't think so. Well, I'm not sure you'd look good with *moobs* anyway," I remarked.

We shrunk back, realizing that Dr. Diane had entered the room at some point and may have heard our conversation. She maintained her professional distance and asked in a perky voice, "How are you feeling?"

"You know—I'm tired, it hurts to pee, and I suck at breastfeeding…. Other than that, I'm feeling great."

"This is your second delivery, so I gather none of that comes as a surprise," she stated, reviewing my chart.

"Not really," I sighed.

"All you can do is make the best of it," she shrugged. "Anything else?"

"Well…now that you ask…there is one thing I've been meaning to ask you about."

Her ears perked up as she looked up from my chart. "Shoot."

"Well, my stomach is really itchy. It's been like this for the past couple of weeks, and I can't figure out why."

I raised my shirt to reveal the red inflammation.

"Oh, sweetie," Dr. Diane said as if she were an old friend. "Those are stretch marks. Nothing you can do about those."

"Son of a bitch!" I exclaimed.

Of course, stretch marks! How could I have been so stupid and not used cocoa butter every day?

"You're so screwed," V remarked.

"There has to be a way to get rid of them," I implored the doctor. "I'm too young to never wear a bikini again…."

"Wait a second," doctor said, bending down to take a closer look at the rash. "I'm sorry to be the bearer of bad news. No wonder you're so itchy. It looks like you've also got a case of PUPPP rash."

"What's *that*?!"

"The exact cause of PUPPP rash isn't known, but the stretching of the skin seems to be a trigger. Nothing you can do about that, either. It'll go away on its own."

Tears formed in my eyes. She regarded me with genuine sympathy until she changed the subject to lighten my mood. I had a hard time following her because I could only think about how hideous I was going to look for the rest of my life and how crazy the itching was making me. She sounded like the *wah-wah-wah* parents' voices in a *Peanuts* cartoon special.

How am I ever going to allow Damien to look at my stomach again? I guess I won't.

"You're cool having sex fully clothed, aren't you, V?"

Crickets.

FORTY

Hotel Sex

CUT TO: *FOUR YEARS AND A TUMMY TUCK LATER.*

Ricky was no longer a baby. He wasn't even a toddler anymore. He had become a hearty, healthy, inquisitive preschooler.

One summer evening, before evening prayers, Damien and I tucked Ricky tightly in bed. I kissed our boy on his forehead and dashed out of the room, leaving my husband in the room to say goodnight.

Why, you may ask? V and I had plans in store. *Big* plans.

It had been a particularly dry week. Between work and the kids' activities, Damien and I hadn't been intimate in over a week, which was quite a lull for us. V and I were beside ourselves.

"Get the socks," V suggested.

"Good idea!"

Allow me to explain. V wasn't referring to argyle, but rather, my white American Apparel thigh high socks with red and blue stripes at the top, which were pretty freaking sexy. I was about to grab the matching booty shorts when V interrupted me.

"No—leave the shorts and the tank. Just the socks!"

"Okay, someone's feeling frisky. Socks it is."

I changed in the bathroom, just in case Damien happened to come upstairs too soon. I sprayed a little perfume on my neck and dabbed a bit behind my ears before tying part of my hair back in a low ponytail.

I know—I'll put on my glasses and read until he stumbles across me.

I positioned myself on our comforter with a book. I propped myself up on a few pillows so that my exposed breasts peeked out over the top of the spine. I immersed myself in *B2B Data-Driven Marketing: Sources, Uses, Results.* Spicy!

Twenty minutes and about fifteen pages later, I heard Damien approach our closed bedroom door. I tensed as the knob handle turned. Unable to contain my excitement, I lowered my book, exposing my breasts.

I gazed seductively across the room as the door swung open. I was about to shout something along the lines of "C'mere, baby!" but unleashed a scream instead.

This is not my husband—it's a mini version of him!

I flung the book across the room while fumbling for cover under the comforter. It was too late; the child's eyes had made full contact on me. I feared he was already scarred for life.

"Mommy, I caught a firefly!" he announced. His expression shifted as he came to a quick realization: "Oh, you're *naked!*"

I need a story—pronto!

"Mommy's *hot*," I improvised. "It's *very hot* tonight. Get out."

I didn't have time to think through the obvious contradiction that, if I were truly hot, I wouldn't be diving underneath the comforter.

Damien, having appeared behind Ricky, seemed at a total loss. "What are you doing?"

Waiting for you to come in here and treat me like a naughty girl. Can't say that!

"I'm reading. It's *very hot* up here! I thought everyone was in bed. *Close the damn door!*"

Ricky chuckled just before Damien managed to shield his hand over the boy's innocent eyes. But the damage was done. My son had seen me naked.

It's going to take years of therapy for him to get over this trauma....

"He couldn't sleep so we went out and caught fireflies," Damien explained.

Why are they still in the bedroom?

"We can talk about this later. Please—put him in bed now!"

"Come on, Ricky," Damien shrugged, turning him around. "Mommy is *crazy*."

That does it. We will never be able to have sex in this house again!

⑥ ⑨ ⑩

I'm sure you now understand why we shifted over to hotel sex at our next opportunity.

We left the boys with their grandparents and set off to Foxwoods Resort Casino in Connecticut for the weekend.

We embarked on the lengthy drive from New Jersey to Connecticut and checked in at the front desk of the hotel. I ducked into the bathroom the instant we entered our room after dropping our bags. I'd been holding in my bladder for a long time during the ride and was pretty desperate.

Once I relieved myself and exited the bathroom, I was greeted by my naked husband sprawled out on the bed.

He caught my surprised expression and asked, "Why wait? We'll be too full after dinner anyway."

"Good point!" I agreed, shedding my clothes.

"No, leave the shirt on!" he commanded.

My shirt was long enough to double as a short dress, which was apparently a big turn-on for him. I did as he suggested and dove on top of him. It felt thrilling to be in a new environment on soft white sheets with the windows open.

Wait—why are the windows open?

"Hey, you forgot to close the curtains!" I protested.

"Karin, we're on the eighteenth floor. No one can see up here.

Not to mention it's all woods around the whole complex."

"Are you sure?"

"Sure, I'm sure. Come on, I'll show you."

He grabbed my hand and walked me over to the window. He placed my hands on the window as we gazed into the sea of blackness. Before I knew what was happening, he slid himself into me.

"*Whoo-hoo!*" V yelped in delight.

I felt like I was in an adult video: *Damien Catches a Fox in the Woods*, starring Karin Freeland. Of course, I knew I'd need to find a better porn name....

⊙ ⊚ ⊚

Whenever I became bored at work, I found myself reliving that sexy night at Foxwoods. I couldn't wait for us to have another getaway— which turned out to be in the Bahamas for our five-year anniversary.

We left the kids with my parents in Rochester for a week and headed off to Sandals. I was a nervous wreck for the first twenty-four hours; we had never been away from the kids this long. I knew the kids would be fine in the care of their grandparents, but I felt big-time mom guilt.

Are the kids too little to leave behind?

It didn't help that I had four messages from my dad when the plane landed. They had taken Ricky to the emergency room for a double ear infection and they needed our consent to treat him. What were the odds of that happening so soon after we left? Once Ricky was prescribed medications and I was given reassurance that he was okay, I was able to relax in the swimming pool with a rum and Coke in hand.

I slid my arms around Damien's back as he gave me a piggyback ride around the main pool. Along the way, he playfully threatened to dunk me and mess up my makeup.

"I noticed you were reading an article on the plane about pleasing your woman," I taunted.

"Yeah, I think I picked up a few good moves," he boasted.

"I'll be the judge of that!"

"As long as I'm in the mood," he countered.

"You mean as long as you don't drink too much and pass out early."

"Exactly!"

We floated around in the water with a few more cocktails until we realized we were turning into prunes. We decided to return to the room and freshen up for dinner.

It took under three minutes for him to be all over me. Something about wet bodies, bathing suits, and a hotel room in the middle of the day really got us going. We made full use of every piece of furniture, taking advantage of the full-length mirror as much as possible.

Throughout our afternoon romp, I looked forward to the moment he was going to break out his new moves. Unfortunately, the moment never came. Don't get me wrong—the sex was great. But I had been expecting some exciting, special twist. I couldn't help but feel a tad bit disappointed.

We showered and dressed for dinner at a hibachi restaurant, where we met with some other couples. They were nice and all but, after dinner, Damien and I found a quiet place to sit outside and watch a thunderstorm in the distance while we enjoyed cigars and beer. (Yes, I had a mini-cigar.)

Something about watching him smoke really tuned me on. His chiseled jaw while puffing away became an aphrodisiac. I nestled up close to him on the hammock for a kiss. We both knew exactly where this was headed.

"We better get back to the room before I can't walk back!" Damien exclaimed.

I could tell from just a quick glance down that it wasn't a gun in his pocket.

We extinguished our cigars and made a beeline for the bedroom.

Night had fallen and all we could hear were the intoxicating sounds of the steel drum band playing down by the main pool.

Damien stepped out onto the patio, where he threw a towel on the chaise lounge and lay down. "Out here?" I asked. "You wanna have sex outside?"

"Why not?" he replied. "We're on the fourth floor. No one can see up here. Even if they can, so what? We'll give them a show!"

"Yeah, why not?!" V roared.

I was putty in his arms. All of the work and mommy stress melted away, and I felt a surge of lust that I hadn't felt in ages.

He was insistent that I straddle him, which was perfect because my feet could touch the floor, giving me leverage for some serious riding motion. A few minutes in—while I was lost in the moment— he hit me with his new move. He twisted my hips about forty-five degrees to the right and thrusted as deeply as he could go.

My jaw opened wide in reaction to the chill skipping up and down up my spine. I arched my back as he repeated the motion. My lengthy hair tickled the inside of his thighs. His thumb found its way to my clit, stimulating it with the perfect amount of pressure and speed. The combo of the friction on my clitoris, his deep penetration, and the beat of the music completely took over my body. My guttural moans—unlike any sounds I'd ever produced—filled the balcony air.

We focused on each other's eyes.

"I love you," he whispered.

And then…*kaboom*—I climaxed! I shoved my face in his chest to muffle my sounds of ecstasy.

Holy shit—he did it! Damien gave me the Big O!

"You mean we did it," V stressed.

She became so overwhelmed by the moment that I think she even shed a tear.

Damien couldn't believe his eyes—or his ears. His pronounced smile widened with pride.

At long last, I was able to let go and surrender control to my primal instincts. I stopped trying to calculate every move, allowing my mind to be fully in the moment.

"*And I thought batteries were expensive,*" I said to V. "*Now we're going to need to splurge for a hotel every time I want an orgasm with him.*"

"*Worth each and every red cent....*"

EPILOGUE

V Gets the Last Word

READ MY LIPS: BEING KARIN'S VAGINA HASN'T BEEN EASY. IT'S SERIOUSLY *dark down here and the climate is unpredictable. One second, it's hot and muggy like a rainforest. The next, it's cold and barren. Now you know why I sometimes come off a bit bitchy.*

It's about time I had a chance to tell my side of the story. Karin is beyond clueless when it comes to her lady parts. She may think she knows what's going on—but she doesn't. She wears suffocating tight jeans and is constantly hacking at me with that Gillette Venus razor. It's a miracle I've been able to hold on to what's left of my abused labia. (By the way: "labium" is singular for one lip; "labia" is plural for both. Karin should have told you upfront this book was going to have lots of educational value.)

Another thing. Why do we always have to explore her idiotic fantasies and not mine? Take the body butter debacle, for example. I know for a fact she's been socking away a tube of Spanish Fly lube in her drawer for ten years. I don't want that crap spritzed anywhere near me. (Here's another piece of important information: Spanish fly is produced by beetles, not flies!)

Anyway, I have my own cool fantasies. Nude beaches, where I can roam free with the ocean breeze in my hair. Afternoon delight twice a month. An extra-large dildo under the Christmas tree might be nice. (I also have a secret Santa fantasy, but that's for another day.)

I guess we've shared some fun, exciting times, too, like when we broke the hotel sink with that college hottie. And, finally, when she got her vibrator collection going. We once came four times in one day. Ah, the good ole days!

Now I'm just sitting around wondering when menopause will hit. Wait a minute, now they tell me I have to worry about perimenopause hitting first. Shit, that can come any day! I'm resigned to my fate as a slab of roast beef on a deli counter.

To get my mind off such morbid things, I like to play pranks on Karin. Sometimes, just when she and Damien are about to get intimate, I drop a little discharge in her underwear for old time's sake. You should see the look of embarrassment on her face!

Anyway, I hope you've enjoyed this inside look at me. Rumor has it that Karin's next literary adventure will be about her breasts—it's a two-volume set.

Hugs and kisses,

V

May 2021

ABOUT THE AUTHOR: KARIN FREELAND

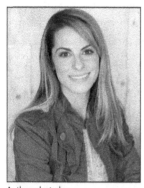

Author photo by
Yolanda Perez Photography LLC

Karin Freeland is an author, speaker, certified life coach, and entrepreneur based in Greenville, South Carolina. Her mission is to help corporate women get unstuck and find their true purpose.

Karin earned her B.S. from the State University of New York, College at Brockport, where she majored in Dance and Business. She spent fifteen years in the most soul-sucking place on Earth, Corporate America, before breaking out to become a full-time author-entrepreneur.

She grew up in Upstate New York and became a Jersey Girl before relocating to South Carolina with her husband—at least until this book comes out—and two boys. She enjoys yoga, online dance classes, and outdoor activities. *The Ins and Outs of My Vagina* is Karin's first book.

Learn more about how Karin transforms women's lives at www. karinfreeland.com/life-coaching.

You can connect with Karin on Instagram @karinfreeland and on Facebook.com/KarinFreelandLifeCoaching.

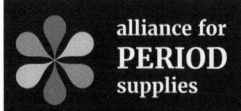

alliance for
PERIOD
supplies

It's that time.

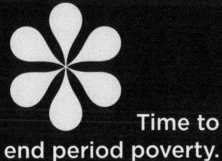

Time to
end period poverty.

A portion of the proceeds
from the sale of my book
will benefit the Alliance
for Period Supplies and help
provide menstrual products
to people in need.

—Karin

CPSIA information can be obtained
at www.ICGtesting.com
Printed in the USA
BVHW081443230921
617401BV00004B/172